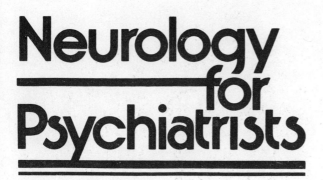

Neurology
for
Psychiatrists

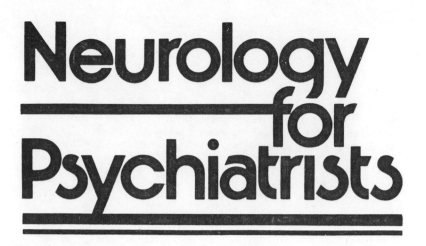

Neurology for Psychiatrists

CHARLES E. WELLS, M.D.
PROFESSOR OF PSYCHIATRY AND NEUROLOGY
VICE CHAIRMAN, DEPARTMENT OF PSYCHIATRY
VANDERBILT UNIVERSITY SCHOOL OF MEDICINE
NASHVILLE, TENNESSEE

GARY W. DUNCAN, M.D.
ASSOCIATE PROFESSOR OF NEUROLOGY
VICE CHAIRMAN, DEPARTMENT OF NEUROLOGY
VANDERBILT UNIVERSITY SCHOOL OF MEDICINE
NEUROLOGY SERVICE
VETERANS ADMINISTRATION HOSPITAL
NASHVILLE, TENNESSEE

 F. A. DAVIS COMPANY, Philadelphia

Library of Congress Cataloging in Publication Data

Wells, Charles E   1929-
   Neurology for psychiatrists.

   Includes bibliographies and index.
   1. Nervous system—Diseases.   2. Psychiatrists.
I. Duncan, Gary W., joint author.   II. Title.
[DNLM: 1. Nervous system diseases.   WL100.3
W453n]
RC346.W44   616.8   79-19972
ISBN 0-8036-9224-2

PREFACE

The purpose of this text is to provide the specialist in one clinical field with a concise summary of what he or she needs to know about another area of clinical specialization. The choice of neurologic topics is selective, because our aim is not to write another comprehensive textbook of neurology but rather to cover the essentials needed for skilled psychiatric practice. The topics chosen are not covered in a comprehensive fashion, but always with an eye toward the particular requirements of the clinical psychiatrist. We seek here specifically to define and provide what the clinical psychiatrist needs to know and will find applicable about clinical neurology. We do not aim to cover all the psychiatric ramifications of neurologic disease, a subject which would fall more appropriately within the purview of the neurologist.

Charles E. Wells
Gary W. Duncan

ACKNOWLEDGMENTS

We wish to express our gratitude: to Doctors James Ellison, Marc Hollender, Fred Plum, and William Webb who have read parts or all of the manuscript and have offered helpful critiques and suggestions; to Dr. George W. Paulson for permission to use several of the Figures in Chapter 2; to Dr. David Drachman, Dr. Cecil W. J. Hart, and the publisher of *Neurology* for permission to use the Figure in Chapter 10; to Mrs. Reba Moore who has effectively and efficiently overseen many details from the inception to the completion of the manuscript; to Anne Dennison, Teresa Prillhart, Patty Shaw, Bettye Stanley and Beverly Steele who have typed and retyped the chapters; and especially to our students whose questions suggested the need for this volume.

C.E.W.
G.W.D.

CONTENTS

CHAPTER 1

INTRODUCTION

Psychiatry and neurology are held together by more than the ties of tradition and the knotty requirements for board certification. They share a primary concern for the brain and its functions and dysfunctions, and thus they share many of the same basic science foundations—neuroanatomy, neurochemistry, neurophysiology, neuropathology, and neuropharmacology. The psychiatrist of today must have a good basic knowledge of these disciplines in order to be able to evaluate behavior and to integrate effectively many of the recent advances in the understanding of psychiatric diseases.

Both psychiatry and neurology are basically medical disciplines; both rely on clinical observations as the primary tool for patient evaluation; both share a primary commitment to the care of people in distress. And most significantly, psychiatrists and neurologists, more often than they generally realize, share the same patients. A great deal of overlap exists in the clinical problems encountered by the two specialties. The neurologist sees a significant number of patients with psychiatric dysfunctions; the general psychiatrist sees a significant number of patients who either have or are suspected to have neurologic disease. In this book we seek to answer some of the psychiatrist's questions about evaluation and management of these patients.

No new ground is broken in this book; rather, it is the outgrowth of changing attitudes in American psychiatry that have been evolving over the past decade. These attitudinal changes have involved not so much a repudiation of the importance of dynamic factors in psychiatric disorders as the recognition that an appreciation of organic factors adds a complementary and sometimes essential dimension to understanding our patients. Neurology and psychiatry, diverging at ever faster rates in the 1940s and '50s, have begun in the '60s and '70s to converge once more in selected areas of mutual concern. This change is seen most clearly in the publication over the past few years of a number of books linking the two disciplines once more. These include two editions of Wells' *Dementia* (1971 and 1977),[9] Pearce and Miller's *Clinical Aspects of Dementia* (1973),[3] Slaby and Wyatt's *Dementia in the Presenium* (1974),[6] two editions of Pincus and Tucker's *Behavioral Neurology* (1974 and 1978),[4] Smith and Kinsbourne's *Aging and Dementia* (1977),[7] and Strub and Black's *The Mental Status Examination in Neurology* (1977).[8] In the same period several books on aging and geriatric psychiatry have also appeared, most seeking as well to link topics of psychiatric and neurologic importance.

The reason the psychiatrist needs a basic knowledge of neurology is not to improve triage function, i.e., so that neurologic problems will be recognized quickly and the patients referred to neurologists. It is naive to believe that the primary reason for a psychiatrist to learn about neurologic disease is to avoid overlooking an organic brain lesion, because there is no convincing evidence that this happens today with any significant frequency. The primary reason that the psychiatrist needs a knowledge of neurology is to enable him or her to provide the best possible care for the identified psychiatric patient with suspected or established coexistent neurologic dysfunction.

In most instances it is artless to believe that the recognition of underlying organic brain disease in the identified psychiatric patient leads to curative treatment by other specialists or implies that further psychiatric treatment is unnecessary. This undeniably occurs, for example, when complete surgical removal of a benign intracranial mass leaves no residual brain dysfunction, or when anticonvulsants abolish bizarre spells that are diagnosed as epileptic. Unfortunately, such examples are rare, and there is little reason to believe that psychiatrists overlook such disorders in significant numbers. Indeed, from a numerical standpoint, there is evidence to suggest that it may be more important for neurologists to learn to recognize and refer patients whose problems are primarily psychiatric. Kirk and Saunders[2] found that 13.2 percent of patients who visited a neurologic outpatient service had primary psychiatric illnesses but of these psychiatric patients, only 13 percent (i.e., thirteen percent of 13.2 percent or 1.75 percent of total patients) were referred for psychiatric evaluation and treatment.

On the other hand, a knowledge of organic brain disease is often important for the psychiatrist in dealing with other physicians. For reasons that are poorly understood, physicians in other specialties occasionally identify a patient's problems as functional in spite of contrary evidence. Engel and Romano[1] remarked on the curious reluctance of internists to recognize and diagnose delirium in their seriously ill medical patients. Saravay and Koran[5] called attention to several situations in which physicians insisted that patients had only functional disease despite clear evidence to the contrary—a patient in whom brain damage

2

had resulted from a fruitless diagnostic procedure, one whose bizarre and destructive behavior frightened the physician, one who failed to respond to treatment that is ordinarily effective, and an abusive and demanding patient who taunted the physician and questioned his competence. The psychiatrist's quick recognition of organicity in these instances protected both the psychiatrist and the referring physician.

We believe that the psychiatrist's need for expertise in neurology goes far beyond the mere recognition of neurologic disease. The psychiatrist needs to study neurology to understand and treat effectively two specific groups of patients commonly encountered in psychiatric practice: (1) patients with primary psychiatric disorders whose symptoms and signs mimic, to some extent, neurologic disease (especially conversion reactions, depressive psychoses, and dissociative reactions); (2) patients whose psychiatric dysfunction coexists with or is secondary to identifiable neurologic disease (especially epilepsy, cerebral trauma, delirium, strokes, and dementia). Although the most difficult differential diagnostic problems arise in the first group, on our services the second group is far more numerous and gives rise to far more therapeutic problems.

The first group is important for two reasons. First, the functional disorders which mimic organic disease are often more easily reversible with treatment than are the organic states they mimic, and thus failure to recognize and treat the functional disorder may prolong the patient's suffering and disability unnecessarily. Second, it is important for the psychiatrist to develop confidence in his or her ability to rule out significant organic disease by appropriate examinations, so that the patient's functional disorder can be treated vigorously and effectively. The psychiatrist who harbors unnecessary doubts that "something organic" has been missed cannot help being a less effective therapist and may limit unnecessarily the treatment modalities employed.

The second group, that is, those whose psychiatric dysfunction coexists with recognized neurologic disease, is notable for the complexity of the clinical problems encountered. These patients do not raise simple either/or type questions for the psychiatrist (i.e., is it psychiatric or neurologic?), rather, they require the psychiatrist to assess the contributions of multiple factors to the production of the patient's symptomatology. For example, a young man has postencephalitic seizures. He is poorly educated because epilepsy is equated with mental retardation in his rural environment, unable to keep a job (in part at least because of his denial of illness), and now is beginning to have trouble with impulse control. What parts do organic disease and dynamic mechanisms play in his past and present difficulties? Another example is a middle-aged man with a long history of "migraine" headaches and declining professional productivity who recently developed seizures with an identified temporal lobe focus and now presents with an acute schizophrenia-like psychosis. In patient after patient such as these, only a thorough knowledge of psychiatric disease coupled with an understanding of neurologic disease will permit a reasonable formulation of the clinical problem. Unfortunately, in many such cases even the most expert psychiatric and neurologic knowledge fails to afford a secure basis of understanding.

REFERENCES

1. Engel, G.L., and Romano, J.: Delirium. A syndrome of cerebral insufficiency. J. Chronic Dis. 9:260, 1959.
2. Kirk, C., and Saunders, M.: Primary psychiatric illness in a neurological out-patient department in north-east England. J. Psychosom. Res. 21:1, 1977.
3. Pearce, J., and Miller, E.: Clinical Aspects of Dementia. Balliere Tindall, London, 1973.
4. Pincus, J.H., and Tucker, G.: Behavioral Neurology, ed. 2. Oxford University Press, New York, 1978.
5. Saravay, S.M., and Koran, L.: Organic disease mistakenly diagnosed as psychiatric. Psychosomatics 18:6, (June) 1977.
6. Slaby, A.E., and Wyatt, R.J.: Dementia in the Presenium. Charles C Thomas, Springfield, Ill., 1974.
7. Smith, W.L., and Kinsbourne, M. (eds.): Aging and Dementia. Spectrum Publications, Inc., New York, 1977.
8. Strub, R.L., and Black, F.W.: The Mental Status Examination in Neurology. F.A. Davis Company, Philadelphia, 1977.
9. Wells, C.E. (ed.): Dementia, ed. 2. F.A. Davis Company, Philadelphia, 1977.

CHAPTER 2

NEUROLOGIC EXAMINATION

Every general psychiatrist should be able to perform a competent neurologic examination appropriate for the patient under consideration. Although the neurologic examination is best learned as a set routine, beyond the learning stage there is no such thing as a routine examination. Each has form and order; each includes certain basic features; but each varies in detail, emphasis, and completeness, the elements of the particular examination being chosen by the physician to suit the needs of the particular patient. The good neurologic examination is, therefore, never merely a duplication of the last but is a special diagnostic procedure designed for a particular patient. The psychiatrist must learn then not only how to perform the individual elements in the examination but also how to select the elements most appropriate for the given patient.

In performing and evaluating the neurologic examination, the examiner must keep in mind that function varies widely in normal persons. Only the Babinski sign is pathognomonic of neurologic disease (involving the corticospinal pathways). Therefore, the examination is not a fishing expedition for pathologic signs but is rather a series of subtle comparisons—comparison of present function with past function, of present function with that observed in other similar persons, of function of one side of the body with that of the other, of function in the upper extremities with that in the lower, of function in the proximal portions of the extremities with that in the distal. The examination described below covers most important features, but it is by no means exhaustive. More detailed accounts are available:[7-9,14,22,26]

The following outline organizes the elements of the examination:
General observations
Mental status examination
Station and gait
Cranial nerve functions

Motor function
Sensory function
Reflexes
Soft neurologic signs
Emergence of primitive responses and reflexes

GENERAL OBSERVATIONS

Observation begins when the physician first encounters the patient and continues throughout the period of history taking and physical examination. Thus it is not set apart from the remainder of the evaluation.

How does the patient present himself to the physician? Is he clean, neatly dressed, and correspondingly well groomed, or is there evidence of neglect and dilapidation? If neglect is present, is it perchance limited to one half of the body? Is the patient's appearance in keeping with his social, economic, educational, and vocational background? Does the patient appear older or younger than his years?

Is the patient alert, responsive, dull, or apathetic? Is he drowsy, unable to attend to the examiner, limited in his attention span? Is he friendly, cooperative, distant, suspicious, guarded, or truculent? Is he uninhibited and indiscreet in discussing topics usually held intimate and private—a frequent observation in organic disorders—or is there evidence that the patient is secretive and withholds information? Is there consistency in the patient's inadequate response to questions? Post[17] stated, "By and large, 'near miss' answers are suggestive of cerebral defects, while 'don't know' answers are more typical of the unwilling and possibly depressed patient." Thus the patient who appears consistently to guess approximate answers to fairly routine questions of fact is more likely to have an organic defect than is the person who answers "I don't know" consistently to the same questions.

Is the patient tremulous, restless, or agitated? Can he sit appropriately for the interview? Are there tremors at rest or other involuntary movements (tics, bizarre gestures, chorea, athetosis)? Are there frequent unconscious movements in the fingers or toes which might suggest loss of postural sense? Are gestures and changes in posture graceful or clumsy? As the patient sits, are there the usual movements of postural readjustment, or is the patient virtually stationary, as occurs with depression and Parkinson disease? Is the face ordinarily expressive, or lacking in animation and masklike? Does he blink more or less than normal? Is there anything notable about his posture? Does he assume the flexed stance of the patient with Parkinson disease? Is one side of the body held in a hemiplegic posture? Does one side move a normal amount while the other is virtually immobile?

Does the patient have obvious difficulty with vision? Is there a squint or use of just one eye at a time (suggesting diplopia)? Does he assume unusual positions in order to see, an observation which might suggest a visual field defect? Do the eyelids droop, close completely with blinking? Is the face symmetrical? Any droop at the corner of the mouth? Is the head erect or tilted?

Is the patient's speech either slow or pressured, of normal volume? Are there articulation defects? Are words used appropriately? Is there groping for words or misuse of familiar words? Does he talk "around" missing words? Is there perseveration or blocking of speech, or disturbance in its rhythm? Are there syntactical errors? Is there any evident difficulty either hearing or understanding the examiner's words?

Obviously much should be learned about the patient's neurologic function from observation alone. The examiner uses the observations as a guide to areas that should be emphasized in the remainder of the neurologic examination.

MENTAL STATUS EXAMINATION

The mental status evaluation is common to both neurology and psychiatry. Much of the data obtained from a formal mental status examination is usually elicited during history taking, and often the drawing out of a thorough history by a skilled examiner obviates the need for a separate, identifiable mental status examination. Most examiners are not so skilled, however, and for them omission of the formal mental status examination is an invitation to error. Strub and Black[23] recently published an excellent short monograph devoted entirely to the mental status examination; we include a number of their suggestions here.

Level of Consciousness

Two aspects of consciousness must be evaluated; (1) level of awareness and (2) level of arousal. The two do not always parallel each other; for example, in delirium one often observes a reduced level of awareness along with a heightened level of arousal (as in an agitated delirium). In recording data about the level of consciousness, it is best to describe the patient's appearance, behavior, and responsiveness in detail (see Chap. 4). The terms ordinarily used to describe these aspects of neural functions—stupor, somnolence, semi-coma, coma—are not precise enough to serve as medical descriptions without further clarifying information.

Orientation

Unless orientation is established without question from the history taking process, it must be proved by exact questioning. One should never simply assume that the alert, cooperative, socially appropriate patient is oriented to time and place. Paulson[15] emphasized how frequently social and affectual preservation mask significant cognitive defects. Do patients know exactly the day, date, time of day, their names, and where they are? Benton, Van Allen, and Fogel[6] reported that neurologists often do not make sufficiently stringent demands for orientation in their patients and thereby fail to recognize the significance of their patients' disorientation. We suspect the same is true for psychiatrists.

Memory

Several aspects of memory must be evaluated in each patient.

IMMEDIATE RECALL

This is usually assessed by the digit repetition test. The patient is asked to repeat digits after the examiner, beginning with three digits and increasing until the patient fails. Digits should be presented at a rate of one each second, taking care neither to group them in rhythmic sequences nor to choose numerals in a natural sequence. The patient is asked first to recall the digits in the order presented by the examiner, then to repeat them backward. Most patients can repeat six or more digits forward and at least four backward.

The patient also may be asked to repeat three unrelated words immediately (testing immediate recall) and then to remember them. Five or ten minutes later the patient is asked to repeat the words again, thus testing recent memory.

RECENT MEMORY

Questions about events in the immediate past usually are used to test recent memory. How did the patient get to the physician's office or to the hospital? If hospitalized, for how long and under what circumstances? What was the last meal, and what was eaten then? What are the names of physicians, nurses, family members, and others who have been in attendance during his illness?

Strub and Black[23] detail several tests which may be used to test visual memory and capacity to assimilate new material, aspects of both immediate and recent memory.

GENERAL GRASP AND RECALL

The patient may be asked to perform a series of increasingly complex tasks: "Raise your right arm." "Put your left index finger on your nose." "Place your right index finger on your left eye." "Put your right index finger on your left ear and your left index finger on your right cheek."

With cerebral disease, the patient's performance often falters as the tasks grow more complex. These tasks depend on the integrity of language functions; they also test for right-left disorientation.

The examiner may read the patient a detail-filled story, asking the patient to recount the story with as many details as possible immediately afterward. Strub and Black[23] offer the following story:

William Stern / a 63-year-old / state representative / from Walton County / Utah / was planning his reelection campaign / when he began experiencing chest pain. / He entered Logan Memorial Hospital / for three days of medical tests. / A harmless virus was diagnosed / and he, his wife / Sandra, / and their two sons / Rick and Tommy / hit the campaign trail again. /

They state that the average patient should be able to produce at least 8 of the 15 relatively separate ideas or information items on immediate recall. Less adequate performance suggests defective verbal recall ability.

REMOTE MEMORY

Can the patient state the date of birth, place of birth, parents' names, schools attended in order, jobs held in sequence, date of marriage, names of children, their ages and order of birth? Can he recall names of presidents who served during his youth, details of important national and local events which took place in the same periods?

Defects in immediate, recent, and remote memory concurrently are characteristics of most cerebral diseases, although immediate recall may be selectively spared in certain amnestic states.

General Intellectual Evaluation

Responses here depend to a significant extent on the patient's educational and past experience. In the sophisticated, well educated patient, intellectual function often is evaluated best through elaborations on the history and the topics covered in the general psychiatric interview. When there is deterioration, however, or when the patient has a scant education or limited intelligence, specific questions are required.

FUND OF INFORMATION

"Who is President of the United States?" "Name the Presidents going backward as far as you can recall." "Who is Vice-President, Governor of your state, Mayor of your city?" "Who represents your district in the House of Representatives?" "Name the senators who represent your state in Congress." "Name five of the largest cities in the United States." "What city is capital of your home state?" "What is the capital of Spain?" "How many weeks make up a year?" "Give an explanation for the seasons of the year."

CALCULATIONS

"Subtract 7 from 100, and then continue subtracting 7 from each sum obtained thereafter." "Multiply 2×4, 6×8, 9×12, 10×11, 12×13." "Divide 12 by 4, 42 by 7, 108 by 12." If errors are committed, does the patient recognize them? Do recognized errors impede further performance?

PROVERBS

Ask the patient to provide an interpretation for several proverbs:
1. People who live in glass houses shouldn't throw stones.
2. The apple falls near its tree.
3. Rome wasn't built in a day.
4. A golden hammer breaks an iron door.

The correctness of a proverb interpretation is usually gauged by the extent of abstraction achieved in the response. However, it must be recalled that concreteness of interpretation is not only a feature of organicity and schizophrenia but perhaps even more often reflects cultural and educational limitations.

SIMILARITIES AND DISCRIMINATIONS

This test requires the patient to explain the basic similarity between two objects or situations and to discriminate between superficially similar details. As in the proverbs test, one is seeking primarily to evaluate the patient's capacity for conceptualization and abstraction.

Ask the patient to describe how the following pairs are similar or alike—a child and a dwarf, a tree and a bush, a river and a canal, a dishwasher and a stove. Ask the patient to explain the difference between a lie and a mistake, idleness and laziness, poverty and misery, character and reputation.

PROBLEM SOLVING

This investigates the patient's ability to deal creatively with challenging but not unusual situations. Ask the patient the following: (1) "If you drove into an unfamiliar city seeking to find a friend who lives there, but you didn't know the address, how would you go about reaching the friend?" (2) "If you got into your automobile one morning planning to go to work but found the car wouldn't start, how would you handle the situation?" (3) "On an icy morning you hear water running under your house, and you suspect that a pipe is broken. What would you do?"

UNDERSTANDING

Does the patient understand his current situation and recognize difficulties that are present and obvious? Does he know that he is ill? Does he believe that nothing is wrong and that all of this attention is unnecessary? Does he understand the cause for and the purpose of the examination? The patient with organic brain disease is often just as out of touch with the reality of the situation as is the patient with schizophrenia or psychotic depression.

LANGUAGE

Language function usually is evaluated most sensitively in the course of history taking and in the remainder of the mental status examination. The physician inquires whether there has been difficulty with speaking, reading, or writing, and listens carefully for dysarthria (difficulty with articulation), dysprosody (interruption of speech melody), problems finding words, errors in choice or use of words, mistakes in syntax, or problems in comprehension. The observer should not accept mistakes too leniently as falling within the range of normal. If history or observation suggests language dysfunction, a more comprehensive examination is required. Specific tests of language function, however, are mainly suitable for amplifying defects that have already been noted. Subtle defects must be picked up by attentive listening during the general portions of the interview.

In carrying out a detailed evaluation of language function, it is best to test for comprehension first, because impaired ability to understand spoken language invalidates or complicates other portions of the examination. First, the patient is asked to point out objects named by the examiner (objects in the room, body parts, articles of clothing). The difficulty can be increased by instructing the patient to point to several objects in correct sequence. Next, the examiner asks a series of increasingly complex questions requiring "yes" or "no" answers. "Is this place a barber (beauty) shop?" "Did you come here by boat?" "Do you eat dinner before going to work in the morning?" Strub and Black[20] pointed out that at least six questions should be asked, because the patient would be expected to guess the right answer to half the questions.

Speech is assayed next by asking for repetition after the examiner of phrases of increasing length. The patient then is asked to name a series of visible objects, body parts, articles of clothing, and colors, and to read aloud a series of printed sentences, some of which may be questions requiring answers (thus testing the patient's comprehension of what has been read).

Last, the patient is asked to write from dictation. Slowness, omissions, and spelling errors are noted.

For the psychiatrist, the aim of detailed evaluation of language functions is the recognition and classification of aphasic defects. The psychiatrist is seldom called on for a fine analysis of aphasia in a patient with diagnosed aphasia, but the psychiatrist should learn to recognize the various presentations of aphasia so that it will not be overlooked. Benson and Geschwind[5] described the three most common types of aphasia encountered clinically, all of which have in common impairment in repeating words and phrases after the examiner. The three types are Broca's aphasia, Wernicke's aphasia, and conduction aphasia; all are caused by lesions in the speech area in the immediate perisylvian region of the dominant hemisphere.

In Broca's aphasia, speech output is sparse and lacking in fluency. Described as "telegraphic," it is made up largely of short phrases lacking articles and prepositions. Comprehension of speech is retained better than is the capacity for speech. Broca's aphasia is due to impairment of function in the motor association cortex of the frontal lobe of the dominant hemisphere (thus accounting for its being called an anterior aphasia). Wernicke's aphasia is characterized by a fluent outflow of speech, often amounting almost to a pressure of speech, but lacking in meaning. Paraphasias and neologisms are common. Comprehension of spoken words usually is severely impaired. Wernicke's aphasia occurs with pathologic involvement of the posterior part of the superior temporal gyrus of the dominant hemisphere, which is the auditory association area (thus accounting for its other name, posterior aphasia). Conduction aphasia is marked by fluent, paraphasic speech (but with more hesitations and pauses than with Wernicke's aphasia), good comprehension of spoken language, and severe difficulty with repetition (as is present to varying degrees in all these varieties of aphasia). Reading for comprehension is also retained in conduction aphasia, which is due most often to a lesion deep in the left inferior parietal region involving the arcuate fasciculus, thus effectively separating the motor from the auditory cortical areas.

Although psychiatrists are seldom called on to treat patients with diagnosed aphasia (despite the frequency of their psychiatric problems[3]), they are not infrequently asked to see patients whose verbal communication is impaired, in association with either a paucity or an excess of verbal production. Thus psychiatric consultation may be requested for the patient who has lost all power of speech.[1] The psychiatrist should know that muteness is rarely a sign of neurologic disease. In acute or massive lesions involving the speech area, the patient may go through a period without speech or any attempts at speech, but this is usually a time when signs of neurologic disability are striking, and thus no diagnostic problem arises. Transient mute periods also occasionally may be a manifestation of a seizure disorder, but careful attention to clinical details almost always reveals signs of other cerebral dysfunction accompanying the muteness. Persistent muteness also is seen in far advanced stages of the cerebral degenerative diseases. When diagnostic problems arise, however, the psychiatrist should recall Benson's statement[3] that "the aphasic is never mute." Muteness is, therefore, usually a manifestation of functional psychiatric disorders—conversion reaction, dissociative reaction, depression, and catatonia. In some of these, the patient makes no effort to speak; in others, the patient makes strenuous and obvious efforts but fails to make a sound or produces only whispers. In aphasic states, on the other hand, the patient almost always tries to speak and usually is able to produce sounds, however incomprehensible they may be.

Psychiatric consultation is requested even more often for patients who speak volubly but incomprehensibly. Although most of these patients will probably be found to be schizophrenic, Gerson, Benson, and Frazier[10] called attention to the problem differentiating the speech of patients with aphasia due to posterior lesions (Wernicke's aphasia) from the speech of schizophrenics. They pointed out that posterior patients tend to respond to questions with shorter answers, are more aware of their communication defects, make obvious efforts to overcome them, and use substitutions in language more than do schizophrenics, whereas schizophrenics often reveal a bizarreness in content that is lacking with posterior aphasias. Benson[4] noted that among patients who have been referred to him for evaluation of "word salad" type of speech, almost all have turned out to have fluent aphasias due to organic brain lesions.

CONSTRUCTIONAL ABILITIES

Tests for constructional abilities have generally been considered more the purview of the psychologist than of either neurologist or psychiatrist. Nevertheless, they are useful for the psychiatrist in the evaluation of patients suspected of either focal or diffuse cerebral disease. Warrington[91] listed six types of tests that demonstrate impaired constructional ability, but for practical purposes most neurologists and psychiatrists limit themselves to asking the patient to copy certain designs and to draw certain objects freehand.

The patient is asked to copy as accurately as possible several designs, either pre-drawn on cards or drawn at the time for the patient by the examiner. These designs commonly include a circle, diamond, cross, and one or two three-dimensional designs (such as a simple box). Other examiners use the familiar Bender designs which are readily available. In the drawing-to-command test, the patient is asked to draw several objects on a blank piece of paper—usually a face, a tree, a clock with hands and numerals, and a house with two sides and roof seen in perspective.

These tasks may be especially useful in nonverbal patients, at times even in patients with recognized language impairment. Good performance in any of these tasks presupposes adequate visual and motor function.

Finally, a thorough mental status examination must include an assessment of mood and an inquiry into possible preoccupations and unusual experiences (obsessions, compulsions, rituals, illusions, delusions, hallucinations). These are a regular feature of every psychiatric evaluation and therefore are not considered in detail here.

STATION AND GAIT

This especially valuable portion of the examination is, unfortunately, often omitted. Subtle disorders of station and gait often pass unnoticed; yet they may provide telltale evidence of focal or diffuse neural dysfunction. Station is evaluated by asking the patient to stand with feet close together, with eyes opened at first, then closed. The patient should then be asked to stand for 10 seconds or so on each foot individually (with eyes opened). Gait is evaluated by asking the patient to walk some distance along a corridor, then to turn about and return. As the patient walks, the examiner notes posture, symmetry of shoulder height, symmetry of arm and leg movements, and rotation of legs and feet. The test is amplified by asking the patient to walk on toes or heels alone, to walk on a narrow line, and to walk heel-to-toe (tandem walk). With experience the physician learns to recognize gaits typical for hemiparesis, cerebellar disease, basal ganglia disease, peripheral neuropathy, and position sense impairment. Gaits which do not conform to these standard patterns suggest a functional etiology. The psychiatrist should also recognize and note less striking evidence of impairment such as general clumsiness, poor coordination, and impaired balance. These manifestations constitute one of the "soft" neurologic signs to be discussed below.

Psychogenic disorders of station and gait are usually manifested by a dramatic and exhibitionistic quality. Even though disability may be profound, the patient often *just* manages to avoid falls and injury, or if the patient does fall, it is in a controlled and protected way. As Weintraub[25] noted, far from indicating disability, movements in functional disorders often actually demonstrate "remarkable ability on the part of these individuals to make rapid and appropriate postural adjustments." In hysterical astasia-abasia (inability to stand or walk), the patient often is able to carry out a full range of motions with full strength when tested in the supine position. Disorders of the cerebellar vermis may be confused with astasia-abasia, for in these disorders (manifested largely by truncal ataxia), dysfunction may be apparent only when the patient sits, stands, or tries to walk. In these patients, however, station and gait abnormalities are typical for cerebellar ataxia and lack the bizarre qualities of astasia-abasia.

14

CRANIAL NERVE FUNCTIONS

CRANIAL NERVE I

Examination of olfactory function by the psychiatrist is called for when a patient complains of impaired smell or taste or when signs or symptoms suggest disease in the frontal fossa. Patency of the nasal passages must be established by examination before testing. Test substances, such as coffee, tea, and tobacco, are used; irritant substances must be avoided because they stimulate pain pathways instead of olfactory pathways.

Each nostril is tested individually while the other is manually occluded. The test substance is held under the nostril, and the patient is told to sniff gently, state if an odor is perceived, and identify the odor if possible.

Many normal people have difficulty recognizing discrete odors, and failure to identify an odor correctly usually merits little attention, so long as the odor is definitely perceived. On the other hand, anosmia is a significant defect, signaling disease along the route of the olfactory nerve.

CRANIAL NERVE II

Evaluation of visual function is an important feature of most neurologic examinations. This includes examination of visual acuity, visual fields, and the optic fundi.

The psychiatrist is not called on to measure visual acuity precisely. The history provides a rough idea of the patient's visual acuity, and it is usually sufficient to learn whether the patient can count fingers, recognize near and distant objects, and read the large and small print on the daily newspaper or a magazine (with each eye separately, with and without glasses).

Visual fields must be tested for each eye separately as well. Lying supine and keeping one eye closed with gentle finger pressure, the patient fixes the open eye on a spot or cross affixed on the ceiling directly over the examining table. The examiner then brings a moving finger from without to within the field of vision in all quadrants, the patient being instructed to indicate when the examiner's finger is first perceived at the periphery. Alternately, the examination may be performed with the patient sitting or standing directly facing the examiner. In this case the patient fixes his vision on the tip of the examiner's nose, and the study is performed otherwise as above.

With practice, the physician learns to recognize "normal" visual fields and to demonstrate slight deviations. This method of visual field evaluation is usually adequate, but if a defect is suspected and cannot be picked up by this method, the patient should be referred to a neurologist

15

or ophthalmologist for perimetry. Homonymous visual fields defects rarely, if ever, result from psychogenic disorders. On the other hand, concentric contraction of the visual fields (tubular vision), characteristically psychogenic in origin, may occur in states of fatigue with poor concentration and, rarely, even in diffuse cerebral disorders.

Ophthalmoscopy allows study of the cornea, lens, vitreous, and optic fundus (disk, retinal vasculature, and retina). The disk is examined especially for color (pallor often indicating optic nerve atrophy), preservation of the optic cup, and clarity of the disk margins. Changes in caliber and state of the arteries and veins are noted, and arteriovenous crossings examined for changes. The veins should be scrutinized for evidence of dilation and for presence of venous pulsations. The retina is scanned for hemorrhages, exudates, and scars.

Well established papilledema is recognized easily, but it is important that the psychiatrist learn to recognize its early, subtle signs: engorgement of veins, loss of venous pulsations, and obliteration of the optic cup. These features require, at the very least, careful follow-up.

Retrobulbar neuritis can cause blindness, yet in the acute stage the fundus may show no abnormality, an observation that sometimes leads to the error of blaming the visual loss on functional disease. It has been described as the condition in which the patient sees nothing and the physician sees nothing. When monocular blindness is due to retrobulbar neuritis, pupillary response to light is usually absent or sluggish bilaterally when light is shined into the blind eye, thus confirming the organic basis for the visual loss.

CRANIAL NERVES III, IV, AND VI

These nerves subserve pupillary size and responsiveness and movement of the eyes and eyelids.

The examiner should observe carefully for drooping of the lid (unilateral or bilateral) and for strabismus, i.e., a lack of parallelism between the visual axes. Pupillary size and shape should be noted, the sides compared, and response to light observed bilaterally when light is shined into each eye alone (the direct and consensual pupillary response). Pupillary accommodation is tested by having the patient fix vision first on a distant object and then on an object several feet away, constriction normally occurring with near vision.

Eye movements are tested by asking the patient to fix gaze on the examiner's finger or on some object held in the hand and then to follow while it is moved to the extremities of gaze in horizontal and vertical planes. The examiner searches for any limitation of conjugate gaze, limitation of movement in one eye, or nystagmus. Convergence is tested by asking the patient to look at the end of the nose or to fix on an object which is then brought nearer in the midline of gaze.

Impaired conjugate gaze in the vertical plane is common in the elderly and, if moderate in degree, should not be considered abnormal. Jenkyn and associates[12] considered limitations in conjugate gaze to be a sign of neurologic abnormality if on upward gaze the deviation of the cornea from midposition were not 5 mm. or more or if on lateral or downward gaze, 7 mm. or more. They considered such limitations in conjugate gaze to be a sign of diffuse brain disease.

Rodin[19] described another abnormality of conjugate gaze which he called impaired ocular pursuit. When lateral conjugate gaze is tested by moving the examiner's finger *slowly* across the visual fields, the eyes normally follow the moving finger smoothly. In some patients, however, this normally smooth pursuit movement is replaced by saccadic movements, the eyes tending to overshoot the target, remain fixed for a brief period, and then advance again ahead of the moving finger. The abnormality can usually be elicited with gaze toward either right or left side; it is not associated with any complaints of visual difficulty. These impaired ocular pursuit movements differ from nystagmus in the lack of slow and fast components and of rhythmicity and in their absence with fixation. The abnormality is not related to vestibulocerebellar dysfunction. Rodin found the sign most consistently in patients with chronic, diffuse diseases of the cerebral hemispheres.

Inquiry should be made as to whether there is any doubling of the image as the object is followed. There are several maneuvers used when diplopia is present to distinguish between the true and the false images, and thereby to determine the paretic muscle or muscles. In practice, however, if there is diplopia without a strabismus which makes identification of the paretic muscle(s) obvious, the psychiatrist should refer the patient for neurologic evaluation rather than trying to work out such a complicated problem unaided.

Except for ptosis, paralytic phenomena involving the extraocular movements are rare in functional psychiatric disorders. Psychogenic ptosis is usually recognized easily by the absence of the compensatory overactivity of the frontalis muscles that is usually present when ptosis is due to a neurologic lesion. On the other hand, spasms of the extraocular and associated muscles are commonly psychogenic in origin, convergence spasm being perhaps most characteristic. Blepharospasm often occurs in basal ganglia disease, however, and should not be mistaken for a functional phenomenon when this is present.

The examiner searches for nystagmus on extreme conjugate deviation of the eyes. Nystagmus is by definition rhythmic and has both a slow and a fast component; it must be differentiated from inability to maintain fixation which is arrhythmic. The former occurs in disease of the labyrinths and vestibular pathways; the latter, in cerebellar disease and with extraocular muscle weakness.

In many normal persons, extreme lateral or vertical gaze provokes fine rapid jerking movements of the eyes. This occurs when the object to be viewed is beyond the effective point of fixation. It is of no pathologic significance and should not be confused with nystagmus.

CRANIAL NERVE V

The fifth cranial or trigeminal nerve has both sensory and motor components. It subserves sensation from the face, forehead, and mucous membranes of the nose, mouth, and tongue. It does not transmit sensory impulses from the posterior half of the cranium or from the ramus of the jaw, often an important point in differentiating sensory loss due to trigeminal nerve lesions from that of conversion reactions. The fifth nerve supplies motor impulses for the muscles that close the jaw and move it from side to side. In practice, sensory abnormalities are much more frequently apparent than is motor loss.

Facial sensation is usually tested both with pin and cotton; the examiner must be certain to check the areas supplied by each of the nerve's three divisions. As in all tests of sensation, the patient's ability to perceive the stimuli is determined first; the patient then is asked to compare the quality of the sensation on the two sides ("Is it equal or different?").

The corneal reflex is elicited by stroking the cornea lightly with a wisp of cotton, approaching the cornea from outside the patient's field of vision to avoid an involuntary blink response. Each eye is tested and the resulting eye blinks compared; the patient is also asked if the stimulus is felt equally on the two sides. This reflex depends on intactness of the sensory fibers of the first division of the trigeminal, its central connections, and the peripheral motor pathways of the seventh nerve; the reflex may be impaired by lesions involving any segment of its route. The corneal reflex is very useful clinically, in part because of its sensitivity to a slight diminution in sensation, in part because it can often be elicited in patients who otherwise are unable to cooperate for the sensory examination (e.g., the stuporous patient).

To test the motor components, the patient is asked to bite down firmly, move the jaw from side to side, and open the mouth. When the patient bites down, the bulk of the masseter muscle on the two sides can be felt and compared, and the bulk of the temporalis muscle assessed at the same time. Jaw movements from side to side are observed for asymmetry and weakness. Because of the configuration of the jaw bone and muscles, a patient with unilateral paralysis of muscles supplied by the fifth cranial nerve can move the jaw forcefully toward the side of motor impairment but cannot move it toward the normal side.

CRANIAL NERVE VII

The physician will already have observed the face for evident impairment of seventh cranial or facial nerve function. Motor function is assessed further by having the patient close the eyes tightly and keep them closed against resistance, elevate the eyebrows and keep them elevated against resistance, and show the teeth. The patient also may be asked to blow out the cheeks, purse the lips, and whistle. Both strength and symmetry are evaluated. Involuntary movements also should be looked for.

The seventh cranial nerve also transmits taste sensations from the anterior two thirds of the tongue. There is seldom a situation that requires the psychiatrist to evaluate this function.

Lesions of the seventh cranial nerve nucleus or the nerve itself result in weakness or paralysis of both the upper and lower facial musculature ipsilaterally. A lesion of the corticobulbar tracts to the facial nucleus usually results in weakness of the lower facial muscles contralaterally, with sparing of the forehead and eyelid muscular functions.

CRANIAL NERVE VIII

The eighth cranial nerve serves both auditory and labyrinthine functions.

Hearing is tested in each ear separately. The external auditory canal must be clear of cerumen. Hearing may be evaluated by measuring the patient's ability to hear whispered or spoken sounds, fingers rubbed against each other, or a vibrating tuning fork (a 128 cps tuning fork is standard). The latter is most easily reproducible. The examiner first sets the tuning fork to vibrating, places its end on the mastoid process, and inquires if the patient hears the sound (to test bone conduction). If so, the patient is asked to indicate when the sound perception is lost, at which time the vibrating end of the tuning fork is placed near the external auditory meatus (to test air conduction). The patient is once more asked if the tuning fork is heard, and if so, to signal the sound's disappearance. The point of disappearance with both bone and air conduction can be measured against the examiner's own perceptions for a rough but usually sufficient appraisal of auditory acuity.

Normally, hearing is approximately equal in the two ears, and normally hearing is better with air than with bone conduction. Unilateral hearing impairment suggests lateralized disease of the middle ear, cochlea, or auditory nerve.

A watch tick is not good for testing hearing, for many normal people, especially the elderly, have some high-tone deafness (the frequency emitted by the ticking watch). The Weber test for the lateralization of sound (well described in standard neurology texts) often raises questions in interpretation even for neurologists and otologists. The psychiatrist will find its use more often confusing than clarifying when dealing with problems of hearing loss.

Labyrinthine dysfunction is often revealed by nystagmus, unusual postures, or ataxia. No specific tests of labyrinthine function are performed in the routine neurologic examination. The procedure for caloric testing is described in Chapter 4.

CRANIAL NERVES IX AND X

These nerves (the glossopharyngeal and vagus) are evaluated through study of the sensory and motor functions of the palate, pharynx, and larynx (although the vagus serves many other parts of the body as well). The patient is asked to open the mouth widely, and any asymmetry of the uvula or palate at rest is noted. The patient is asked to say "ah," and the elevation of the palate and constriction of the pharyngeal muscles are observed. The examiner then touches the posterior pharyngeal wall on the left and right sides with a swab or tongue blade, looking for the reflex contraction of the pharyngeal musculature (the gag reflex) and asking about the patient's perception of the stimuli.

The examiner looks especially for drooping of one side of the palate or impaired contraction of the muscles on one side of the pharynx. Such asymmetries often result from peripheral nerve lesions. Bilateral weakness of these muscles, on the other hand, often occurs with bilateral corticospinal tract disease and with myasthenia gravis.

The presence or absence of the gag reflex per se has been much overrated as a clinical sign. Although present in most people, many normal persons lack a gag reflex, and its absence should not be considered pathologic. If the patient perceives the stimulus on the posterior pharyngeal wall and is able to elevate the palate and constrict the pharyngeal muscles at will, the absence of the gag reflex is of no significance.

More complex functions of the ninth and tenth nerves can be evaluated by observing the patient's ability to swallow or to drink water and by noting the quality of the voice.

CRANIAL NERVE XI

This nerve innervates the sternocleidomastoid and trapezius muscles. The sternocleidomastoid muscle acts to turn the head away from the side of the muscle, i.e., the right sternocleidomastoid turns the head to the left. One-sided weakness of the sternocleidomastoid muscle thus impairs ability to turn the head toward the other side. When unilateral weakness results from a conversion reaction, however, the patient often is unable to turn the head toward the affected side.

The trapezius muscle, which elevates the shoulder and braces it backward, is innervated only in part by the eleventh cranial nerve, and texts differ as to whether the upper or the lower portion is innervated by this nerve. Its strength can be evaluated rapidly by testing both functions against resistance.

CRANIAL NERVE XII

This motor nerve innervates the tongue, which should be observed first at rest with the mouth open. Atrophy and/or fibrillations of the tongue at rest suggest lower motor neuron disease. The patient then is asked to protrude the tongue in the midline. With unilateral weakness, the tongue protrudes toward the side of the weakness instead of its usual midline position. Weakness of the tongue without atrophy usually results from an upper motor neuron (corticobulbar) lesion. Thus a lesion involving the motor pathways descending from the right hemisphere to the left side of the brain stem causes weakness of the left half of the tongue, with deviation of the tongue toward the left on protrusion.

MOTOR FUNCTION

Motor function is evaluated both by observation and by specific testing. The extent of the examination varies widely, depending largely on history and preceding observations. Assessment proceeds in an orderly manner, with motility of the cranium, neck, arms, trunk, and legs evaluated in succession. When motor impairment is a complaint, however, it may be better to examine the symptomatic region first.

Observation

In addition to the features already mentioned, skeletal and muscular development must be assessed. Shortness of a limb or smallness of one hand or foot may follow cerebral damage in early life. The examiner looks for evidence of muscle wasting, which in its early stages is likely to be most discernible in the muscles of the hand and in the anterior tibial region of the legs. Small degrees of muscle atrophy are usually more easily recognized by observation than by exact measurement. Muscle bulk is compared on the two sides of the body and between the proximal and distal portions of the extremities. The examiner also searches for fasciculations (irregular, involuntary, arrhythmic, asymmetric contractions of small groups of muscle fibers), often an indication of lower motor neuron disease. Fasciculations can be identified with certainty only when the patient is completely relaxed in a warm examining room.

Examination

RESISTANCE TO PASSIVE STRETCH

Muscle tone, the resistance felt when the extremities are manipulated in the relaxed patient, can be evaluated by moving the wrists, elbows, shoulders, hips, and knees through a full range of motion. The appreciation of normal muscle tone is based on subjective experience and can be learned only by practice. With practice, however, the physician gets the feel of normal resistance to passive movement and learns to distinguish those changes due to disease from those due to faulty relaxation.

A reduction in resistance to passive stretch may be seen with cerebellar disease, lower motor neuron lesions, and primary muscle disease, and is an observation usually of limited diagnostic assistance. Increased resistance to passive movement, on the other hand, is often valuable diagnostically.

Two types of increased tone are usually described: "clasp knife" and "lead pipe," or spasticity and rigidity respectively. With spasticity, the resistance is usually greatest just after muscle stretch begins, but, as it continues, resistance gives way abruptly with full displacement of the part following. Clasp knife spasticity is characteristic of corticospinal tract disease. With lead pipe rigidity, resistance is uniformly increased throughout the rage of motion, a characteristic of extrapyramidal tract disease. The "cogwheel" rigidity of Parkinson disease consists of rigidity with a superimposed tremor. Increased resistance to muscle stretch must be differentiated from increased resistance due to contraction of joints which is frequent in patients immobilized for long periods.

A less well recognized increase in resistance to passive movement is paratonic rigidity (involuntary rigidity, gegenhalten, negativism). It is appreciated as an irregular catching felt in opposition to the examiner's movements after the patient has been instructed to relax. Paulson[15] noted that it may become more obvious if the manipulation is performed impatiently while the patient is urged rather sharply to relax. Paratonic rigidity is frequently a sign of diffuse brain disease. Jenkyn and associates[12] described a variation in which the examiner suddenly withdraws support from the manipulated extremity. The extremity normally drops abruptly. Any delay is called abnormal limb placement, another sign of diffuse brain dysfunction.

Muscle strength is evaluated by testing for maximal power of movement at the shoulders, elbows, wrists, fingers, hips, knees, and ankles, in that order. When testing strength, the examiner should palpate the contracting muscles as well as assess the force of the contractions. In this way the jerky, poorly sustained contractions characteristic of cerebellar disease may be appreciated, as may the sudden "giving way" in patients with weakness due to functional disorders. Palpation also may reveal the simultaneous contractions in agonist and antagonist muscles common in psychogenic weakness. When circumscribed weakness is established, evaluation of individual muscle function may be in order. The psychiatrist usually should refer the patient to a neurologist when such detailed evaluation is required.

In evaluating weakness, most examiners ask three basic questions:
1. Is the weakness circumscribed, involving only one or a few muscle groups?
2. Does the weakness involve the two sides of the body symmetrically or asymmetrically?
3. Is the weakness more severe proximally or distally?

Weakness limited to one or a few muscle groups is usually due to anterior spinal root or peripheral nerve disease. Weakness limited to one side of the body most often is due to a lesion of the cerebral hemispheres. Symmetrical weakness on the two sides of the body is most often secondary to spinal cord disease, anterior horn cell disease, peripheral neuropathy, or muscle disease. Symmetrical distal weakness is characteristic of peripheral neuropathy; symmetrical proximal weakness, of primary muscle disease.

Mild to moderate diffuse muscle weakness is usually of little neurologic importance. Muscles weak from any cause may fatigue rather quickly with repetitive movements. Only with myasthenia gravis, however, does repetition induce paralysis, except in certain cases of psychogenic weakness. In others with psychogenic weakness, repetition of movement along with verbal encouragement may actually result in increasing strength.

In evaluating strength and motility, observation of the patient's behavior may be as useful as test performance. Obvious lack of effort carries implications that require further investigation, as does a theatrical display of excessive effort. When this is present alongside weakness or dysmetria, a psychogenic origin for the impairment is usually implied. Most patients with significant weakness or impaired motility are appropriately worried about their condition. Apathy or lack of concern are significant observations, the former often accompanying depression, the latter conversion reactions. Excessive concern over relatively trivial dysfunction requires equal attention.

Several other observations may be especially useful to psychiatrists who are often called on to evaluate patients whose weakness is suspected to result from a conversion reaction. In unilateral weakness of psychogenic origin, the muscles of the face and tongue and the platysma and sternocleidomastoid muscles are usually spared (except that the patient may have weakness turning the head *toward* the hemiparetic side [vide supra]). With psychogenic hemiplegia, the patient may be unable to adduct the paretic arm or leg on command, but if these are placed in the adducted position bilaterally and the patient asked to maintain this position against resistance, adductor contractions can usually be observed and palpated on the hemiplegic as well as the normal side (because it is difficult to adduct the normal extremity voluntarily without also contracting the corresponding muscles on the weak side). In psychogenic paraplegia, there is usually no dysfunction of the sphincters.

In cases of suspected psychogenic weakness, it is important to test strength with the patient in different positions. It is not unusual, for example, to observe striking weakness in a muscle group with the patient supine which abates or disappears when the patient is tested in a standing position, and vice versa.

When a normal person in a supine position flexes one thigh and lifts the leg, there is a downward movement of the other leg, easily felt by placing one's palm beneath the heel. In cases of psychogenic weakness, this phenomenon is absent in the normal leg when the patient attempts to raise the paretic one, although the downward movement may be felt in the paretic one when the patient raises the normal one. This is the classic Hoover's sign—one of many specifically described for the detection of psychogenic weakness. The interested reader is referred to De-Jong's text for other such maneuvers.[8] These signs and maneuvers are often of some help when weakness is profound and the patient is unsophisticated, but the observations are likely to be much less definitive in instances of milder impairment in more sophisticated subjects.

COORDINATION

Coordination may be tested in many ways, but only a few are necessary for most psychiatric patients. Both rapid rhythmic and fine movements should be assessed, in both extremities, separately and together, the latter to evaluate the integration of movements between the two sides.

The patient may be asked to perform any or all of the following acts rapidly and repetitively: to pat the hand, tap the feet, open and close the fist, alternately pronate and supinate the extended arm, oppose the thumb and index finger, or slap the palm and the back of the hand alternately on the thigh. Performance on these tests for rapid, rhythmic, alternating movements may be impaired significantly even when the strength is normal.

More exact movement is tested in the upper extremities by asking the patient to touch a distant point with the index finger, return the index finger to the tip of the nose, and then move back and forth quickly and accurately between the two points. In the lower extremity the patient, in the supine position, is asked to lift the leg and touch the examiner's index finger repetitively with the great toe, as the examiner shifts the position of the target finger in space. Tests of fine coordination include evaluation of patient's ability to write, draw, copy designs, drink from a cup, or simulate eating from a fork. Tests for coordinated use of both arms and both legs include asking the patient to clap the hands together, button and unbutton clothing, transfer an object back and forth rapidly from one hand to the other, simulate kicking a ball, and hop first on one foot and then the other (in addition to the evaluation of gait).

As the patient goes through these acts, the examiner looks for clumsiness, slowness, imprecision, ataxia, failure to alternate movements successfully, and breakdown in order of sequential movements. In those actions requiring fine cooperation between the two sides of the body, the examiner observes any lack of grace, clumsiness, or overt failure of coordination.

INVOLUNTARY MOVEMENTS

The physician looks for involuntary movements such as tic, chorea, athetosis, tremor, myoclonic jerks, or focal seizures. Patients sometimes become skillful in concealing involuntary movements by melding them into apparently purposeful acts, and the examiner must be alert to this possibility in patients who are restless and fidgety. In assessing involuntary movements, it is important to note whether they are present at rest and with movement, whether they disappear with movement, and whether they can be suppressed, even temporarily, at will.

SENSORY FUNCTION

For a reliable examination, the patient must be alert, able to participate, and cooperative. It requires the examiner to be patient, skillful, and perhaps a bit skeptical of the patient's responses. Ideally, the sensory examination should be brief. Few patients can respond accurately for a long examination, and if such is necessary, it is preferable to perform it in several sittings.

Not every patient requires a complete sensory examination. It is usually sufficient to test for appreciation of cotton and pin over the face, hands, and feet; passive movement in the fingers and toes; and two-point discrimination on the finger tips. A more detailed examination is indicated if abnormalities are uncovered by these basic tests or if any of the following are present:

1. Complaints of numbness, pins-and-needles, tingling, pain, or hyperesthesia
2. Trophic skin changes, unnoticed burns and other evidence of suspected trauma, or painless ulcers
3. Pseudoathetosis (small groping movements of the fingers and toes frequently associated with diminished position sense)
4. Ataxia
5. Evidence pointing to a lesion of the brain stem or cerebral hemispheres.

As with other neurologic functions, sensory loss is seldom absolute; sensory changes are more likely to be subtle and qualitative. Again, sensation on one side of the body is compared with the other, and the distal parts of the extremities with the proximal. When a sensory defect is identified, it is best to delineate the area by moving the test stimulus *from* the area of abnormal perception *to* the area of normal function rather than the other way.

Aberrations in the sensory examination should not be accepted as valid unless the findings can be replicated with some ease. Inconsistency should cause the examiner to question the conclusions that can be drawn from the observations rather than to suppose the examination was lacking in skill.

The examiner is concerned with the patient's reaction to the testing procedure as well as with the responses themselves. Patients with psychogenic disorders of sensation vary in their reactions to sensory testing, but their reactions usually differ from those of patients with purely neurologic impairment. Some appear indifferent to sensory losses which would be seriously threatening to the normal person; others appear indifferent to stimuli evoking what they describe as sensations of excruciating pain. Still others writhe in discomfort with the least noxious of stimuli, at the same time having none of the physiologic accompaniments of pain.

Psychiatrists should be familiar with certain patterns of sensory loss that are characteristic of psychogenic disorders. Abrupt borders for zones of sensory impairment are rare in organic disease; thus a well defined, abrupt border between an area of analgesia and one of normal perception suggests a psychogenic disorder. Normal perception of other sensory modalities within an area of total anesthesia to pinprick has the same connotation. Unilateral sensory loss with a discrete midline border is likewise unusual in organic lesions, and if the midline border includes the penis, vagina, and rectum, the likelihood of organicity is further reduced. If there is midline loss of vibratory sense over the sternum and skull, there can be no organic explanation. The psychiatrist must keep in mind, however, that conversion reactions are not unusual with organic brain lesions, so that the presence of one does not rule out the other.

Specific Modalities

PAIN

Pain perception is tested by pinprick. The stimulus must be easily recognizable as a pinprick yet not so painful as to induce withdrawal. Normal patients perceive the stimuli as sharp, equal on the two sides, and equal proximally and distally in the extremities. If there is reason to question the patient's reliability, point and head of the pin should be used as stimuli in random sequence and the patient instructed to identify the "point" or "head" after each stimulus.

TOUCH

Touch is tested with a wisp of cotton drawn lightly for a centimeter or so across the patient's skin. The patient is instructed to close the eyes and respond each time the stimulus is felt. Touching hairs results in more sensory input than touching skin alone, a factor to be taken into account when evaluating the patient's responses. Again, the patient is asked to compare the quality of the sensation in symmetrical body parts, proximally and distally.

TEMPERATURE

Temperature appreciation rarely need be evaluated by the psychiatrist. It can be tested by having the patient distinguish between tubes of hot and cold water and by asking the patient about the intensity of the temperature perception. From a practical standpoint, if the case is so complicated that temperature testing is required for its clarification, the patient probably should be referred to a neurologist for definitive evaluation.

PASSIVE MOVEMENT

This is tested by movement at the distal interphalangeal joint of the index finger and at the interphalangeal joint of the great toe (Fig. 2-1). The digit is immobilized except for the distal phalanx which is grasped at its *sides* between the examiner's thumb and index finger. The patient is asked to report the direction of each movement, whether up or down. Again, no exact standards of normality exist, but with practice the examiner quickly learns to distinguish significant impairment.

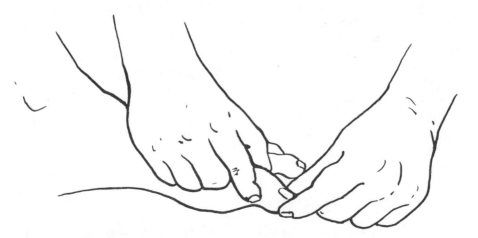

FIGURE 2-1. Correct method for testing passive movement sense.

POSITION SENSE

Impaired position sense and passive movement appreciation usually, but not always, occur together, so that it is generally unnecessary for the psychiatrist to test both. Position sense can be tested specifically by asking the patient to close the eyes. The examiner then moves the patient's hand or foot to various positions in space and asks the patient either to touch the positioned index finger with the free index finger or to point to the positioned heel.

VIBRATORY SENSE

This is usually assessed by measuring how long a vibrating 128 cps tuning fork is perceived when the fork is pressed against bone distally in the upper and lower extremities. Decreased vibratory sense in the ankles and feet is common in old age and, thus, should not be accorded pathologic significance unless severe.

CORTICAL SENSORY FUNCTION

Several tests are available to measure those sensory modalities dependent upon the sensory cortex. The psychiatrist should be skilled in the use of some of them. Cortical sensory functions require that the pathways which transmit touch from the periphery to the cortex be intact; thus evaluation of cortical sensory functions is difficult when touch is impaired.

Two-point discrimination is an excellent and quantifiable test of cortical function. Most normal persons can distinguish two points touching the finger pads when they are separated by 5 mm or more (and many can distinguish two points at even less distance). It is important that the points be dull so that pain pathways are not activated. The test is of greater value in comparing one side with the other than in determining the absolute distance of discrimination.

Graphesthesia, the ability to recognize numbers or letters traced with a blunt object on the pads of the finger tips, palms, or legs, is another cortical sensory function. Once more, a comparison of function between the two sides is more useful than a determination of the absolute size of the letters of figures recognizable.

Other useful tests of cortical sensory function include the recognition of objects (coins, paper clip, button, safety pin) and textures (silk, cotton, wool, steel wool) placed in the hand and manipulated by the patient. A difference in ability on the two sides is again more useful in general than is bilateral difficulty. The ability to recognize slight differences in weight of equal-sized objects placed in the two palms is another approach, as is the ability to appreciate double simultaneous touch or pin stimuli. In this test, a patient is touched randomly either unilaterally or bilaterally at symmetrical locations, and the patient is asked to report whether the stimulus is perceived on one or both sides. Consistent failure to appreciate stimulation on one side with bilateral stimulation (unilateral neglect, inattention, or extinction) is evidence suggesting dysfunction of the opposite cortex.

REFLEXES

Both muscle stretch reflexes and superficial reflexes are important. Muscle stretch reflexes (also called tendon jerks) result from a sudden stretching of the muscle and usually are evoked by tapping the muscle tendon. Superficial reflexes are evoked by stroking the skin. Muscle stretch reflexes are characteristically segmental; superficial reflexes usually involve more than a segmental level of the spinal cord (i.e., they are multisynaptic).

Muscle Stretch Reflexes

Muscle stretch reflexes may be elicited with the patient either seated or supine, but the patient must be well relaxed whatever the position. The limb is positioned so that the muscle to be tested possesses a mild degree of passive tension. The reflex can be evaluated more accurately if the examiner palpates the muscle and feels the actual response rather than relying on visual observation of the accompanying displacement of the part. Palpation is particularly useful in evaluating the biceps and the quadriceps reflexes. Minor but clinically important asymmetries are often brought out by the examiner's using the least stimulus possible rather than employing a uniformly vigorous stimulus.

The following muscle stretch reflexes are sought in the usual neurologic examination (with corresponding spinal segments given in parentheses):

Biceps (C5, C6)
Triceps (C7)
Forearm supinator (C6, C7)
Forearm pronator (C8, T1)
Quadriceps (knee jerk) (L3, L4)
Ankle jerk (obtained by tapping the Achilles tendon to produce stretching of the gastrocnemius and soleus muscles) (S1, S2)

The muscle stretch reflexes are usually estimated on a 0 to 4+ scale, but because these are subjective evaluations, the level assigned varies from examiner to examiner. Asymmetries in the muscle stretch reflexes are usually more important than their briskness. Some normal subjects have vigorous muscle stretch reflexes; a few are areflexic. Hypoactive lower extremity reflexes are common in the elderly.

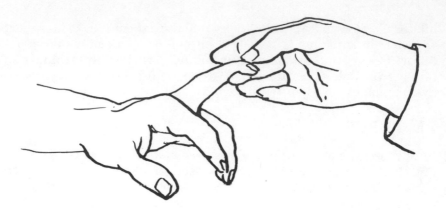

FIGURE 2-2. Testing for Hoffmann sign.

HOFFMANN SIGN

Another reflex often sought is the flexation of the thumb and fingers which sometimes follows flicking the nail of the extended middle finger while the other fingers are pronated and relaxed in the flexed position (Fig. 2-2). When this occurs, the patient is said to have a Hoffmann sign. This is often present with corticospinal tract disease but may occur as well when muscle stretch reflexes are brisk from any cause. The sign also often appears bilaterally with diffuse brain disease. The Hoffmann sign is not necessarily pathologic, but it is often helpful clinically, especially when it is asymmetrical.

ANKLE CLONUS

Ankle clonus must be sought whenever the muscle stretch reflexes are brisk to hyperactive. To elicit ankle clonus, the ankle must be kept as relaxed as possible and the knee, partially flexed. The examiner briskly dorsiflexes the foot and maintains pressure on the sole of the foot (Fig. 2-3). Correct performance of this maneuver requires practice, but it should be learned by all psychiatrists. If rhythmic, repetitive flexion movements of the foot result, ankle clonus is said to be present. Sustained ankle clonus is a sign of upper motor neuron dysfunction, but the significance of lesser degrees of clonus is unclear. Clonus of psychogenic origin has been described, especially with anxiety; it is usually arrhythmic and poorly sustained. In the rare instance in which ankle clonus of psychogenic origin is sustained, it may fail to be abolished by brisk plantar flexation, a maneuver that aborts clonus of neurogenic origin.

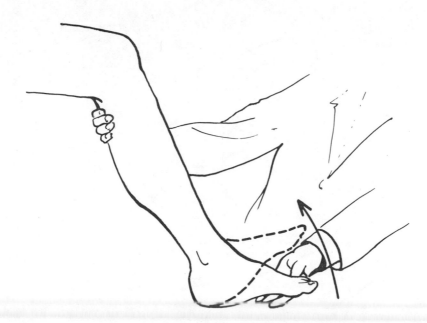

FIGURE 2-3. Maneuver for eliciting ankle clonus.

Superficial Reflexes

SUPERFICIAL ABDOMINAL REFLEX

This reflex is elicited by stroking the abdomen lightly with a blunt point (a key is often satisfactory), making certain that the stimulus does not cause pain. The skin is stroked from the flank toward the midline in the direction of the dermatome distribution (Fig. 2-4), in both upper and lower abdominal quadrants, bilaterally. Normally this results in a brisk reflex contraction of the abdominal muscles on the side stimulated. Both strength and symmetry of the reflex are noted.

The superficial abdominal reflexes can be elicited in most normal people, although practice is required to obtain them predictably. The reflex usually persists into old age. Often it cannot be detected clinically in patients with pendulous abdomens, whether due to multiple operative procedures or extreme obesity. The reflex is often diminished or absent in upper motor neuron disease. Thus it may be weak or absent unilaterally with unilateral corticospinal tract lesions, bilaterally with bilateral corticospinal tract disease.

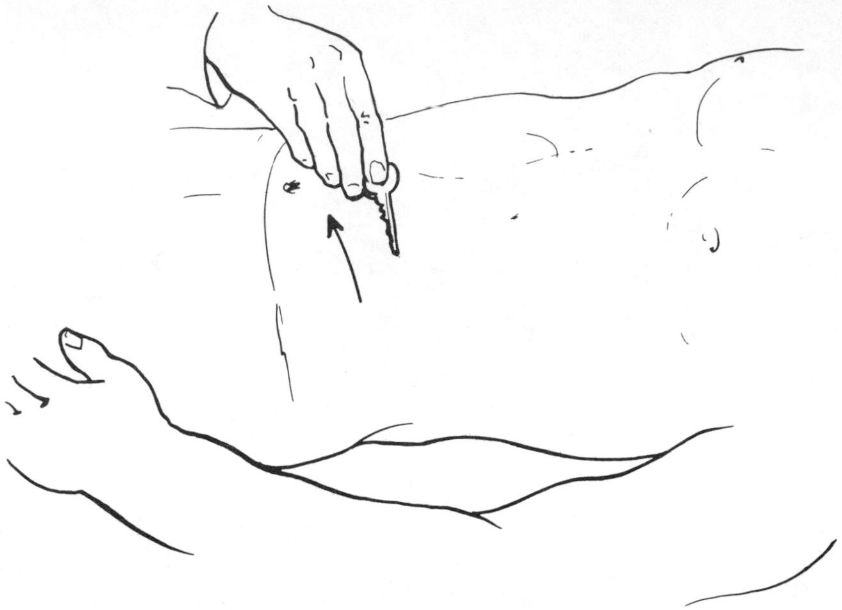

FIGURE 2-4. Correct method for eliciting abdominal reflex.

CREMASTER REFLEX

A similar reflex is the contraction of the cremaster muscle, raising the testis, that follows stimulation of the skin on the inner aspect of the upper thigh. This reflex, too, usually is diminished or absent on the side affected by corticospinal tract disease and bilaterally with a cord lesion at or above the level of T12 or L1 affecting the corticospinal tracts bilaterally. This reflex is less predictable and thus less useful clinically than the superficial abdominal reflex. It is likely to be specifically useful to the psychiatrist only in cases of sexual dysfunction in which there is a question of organic impairment.

RESPONSE TO PLANTAR STIMULATION

This response is brought forth by stroking the sole of the foot with a blunt point, moving the object from the heel toward the ball of the foot along its lateral border and then inward (Fig. 2-5). Most psychiatrists will do best to observe only for the resulting movement of the great toe at the metatarsophalangeal joint. The normal response is a slow, definite plantar flexion of the great toe. The abnormal response, i.e., the Babinski sign, is usually a somewhat more rapid dorsiflexion at the same joint. The response is not always clearcut. Sometimes repeated stimulation and meticulous observation is required before the examiner

32

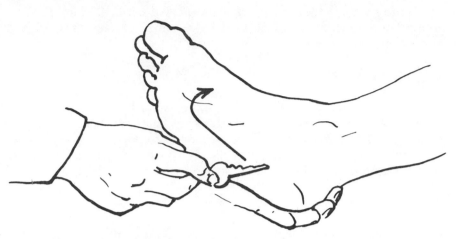

FIGURE 2-5. Direction of stroke to elicit plantar reflex.

can make an interpretation, and in rare cases a definitive interpretation may be impossible. In the adult, the Babinski sign, i.e., unequivocal dorsiflexion, is always pathologic, diagnostic of corticospinal tract disease. A number of alternative maneuvers to plantar stimulation have been described. In general they are less sensitive indicators of neural dysfunction, resulting from a widening of the reflexogenous zone.

SOFT NEUROLOGIC SIGNS

So far we have dealt only with the conventional neurologic examination as it might be tailored to the needs of the practicing psychiatrist. Over the years, however, investigators have sought ways to detect evidence of neurologic disease that cannot be picked up by conventional examinations. Patients have been studied who have disorders for which there is at least some cause to suspect an underlying neuropathologic substratum, disorders such as mental retardation, learning disabilities, behavior disorders, and hyperkinesis. In studying these and related disorders, a number of observations have been made which suggest an underlying failure of neural integration. These observations have come to be called "soft" neurologic signs, the name implying that although they do not predict specific lesions, they nevertheless suggest a possibility of neurologic dysfunction, and that when these soft signs are clustered in an individual patient, they suggest the likelihood of an organic abnormality. In recent years, the search for soft signs has included patients with conventional psychiatric diagnoses. In these investigations, Rochford and associates[18] have defined a neurologic abnormality as the presence in any patient of two or more soft signs.

A large number of these soft signs has been described. Those considered below are included because the tests are in general easy to perform, and the observations easy to evaluate.

Speech Defects

The speech defects for which the examiner listens here are not those of frank neurologic disease as described above. These are more subtle and more difficult to describe. The examiner listens for such things as hesitancy, minor articulatory defects, dysrhythmic speech, defects in breath regulation, and occasional stuttering.

Abnormal Motor Activity

Hypokinesis, hyperkinesis, excessive restlessness, choreiform movements, snorts and gutteral sounds—in short, evidence that the patient cannot sit quietly and at ease—may be evidence of neurologic impairment.

Disturbances of Balance and Gait

Most persons maintain a standing posture easily, walk with a certain grace and fluidity, and turn without unsteadiness. In this regard, the examiner looks for unsteadiness of stance, clumsiness, lack of grace or rhythm in walking, poor balance with change of direction, and significant difficulty when the patient is asked to walk a narrow line, tandem walk, or stand on one foot.

Cranial Nerve Abnormalities

The defects in cranial nerve function identified as soft neurologic signs are the sort that would get only cursory notice in the routine examination—a slight anisocoria or esotropia, mild ptosis of one eyelid, and minor flattening of one nasolabial fold are examples.

Abnormalities of Motility

MOTOR IMPERSISTENCE

Most normal persons are able on request to maintain a fixed posture and to sustain a steady muscle contraction for a significant period of time. Certain patients with maturational defects and with central nerve system disease cannot do so. This inability is called motor impersistence.

Joynt, Benton, and Fogel[13] studied the phenomenon of motor impersistence and described nine tests for eliciting the phenomenon, among them:

Close your eyes and keep them closed. (20 secs.)

Stick out your tongue and keep it out. (20 secs.)

Open your mouth and keep it open. (20 secs.)

Take a deep breath, say "ah" softly and sustain the tone as long as possible. (18 secs.)

In parentheses are the minimum times the subject is expected to maintain the act. Motor impersistence, rare in normal children or adults, has been reported to correlate best with bilateral cerebral disease or with pathology limited to the right hemisphere, but one wonders if aphasia may not preclude testing patients with comparable damage to the left hemisphere. Tests for motor impersistence may also bring to light involuntary movements, especially choreiform movements, which may be masked by the patient in other circumstances.

COORDINATION DEFECTS

Maneuvers to bring out coordination defects have already been described. Coordination defects that are considered soft neurologic signs are less clearcut than gross ataxia; rather they encompass a certain clumsiness and ungainliness, jerkiness, or difficulty achieving mutuality and reciprocity in acts involving left and right extremities. Not everyone lacking in grace has a coordination defect, but ungainliness of an unusual degree should be noted and should suggest the possibility of neurologic dysfunction.

MIRROR MOVEMENTS

Mirror movements (unconscious, symmetrical, adventitious movements lesser in amplitude appearing in the opposite extremity with volitional movement of the other extremity) are common in childhood and disappear with maturation. They may persist in patients with neonatal cerebral damage or other disturbances in cerebral development. Later in life they often reappear after unilateral cerebral damage. The patient who develops left hemiparesis, for example, may display mirror movements of the left hand when a fist is made volitionally with the right.

Abnormalities of Sensation

GRAPHESTHESIA AND STEREOGNOSIS

Tests for two-point discrimination, identification of numbers and letters traced on the skin, and recognition of objects, textures, and weights were described above. Unilateral defects in these functions are regarded as hard neurologic signs indicating focal brain disease. When the difficulty is bilateral, however, and not so much severe loss of the capacities as a raised threshold for their appreciation, this is considered a soft sign, and its significance is less exact.

DOUBLE SIMULTANEOUS STIMULATION

One method of testing with double simultaneous stimulations has been described above, the method most useful for identification of focal defects (a defect usually considered a hard sign). By another method, the face (cheek) and either the ipsilateral or the contralateral hand are touched simultaneously by the examiner's fingers. The subject is asked to specify the number of fingers felt and their location. If only one is reported, inquiry is made to see if the second stimulus might have been felt but not reported. The test is repeated 10 times if the patient fails to identify the two stimuli correctly in the initial trials.[2] Errors are common initially even in normal subjects, but once the normal subject catches on, there are virtually no more errors. Errors are usually of two types: failure to perceive the hand stimulus or displacement of the hand stimulus to the face. Children below the age of seven are unable to perform this task. Errors are common in diffuse organic brain disease, and the organic patient often cannot learn to do the task even with repeated efforts.

REFLEX CHANGES

Bilaterally symmetrical hyperreflexia or hyporeflexia (of the muscle stretch reflexes) has been considered by some to be a soft neurologic sign. We have observed so much variation in reflexes in normal subjects, however, that we doubt if this should be considered even a soft sign of organic dysfunction.

EMERGENCE OF PRIMITIVE RESPONSES AND REFLEXES

Several reflexes present in the fetus, neonate, and young child disappear in the process of normal growth and development. Some of these have been observed to emerge again later in life in conjunction with cerebral disease.[16] Demonstration of these reflexes, especially if several are present in the same patient, is often helpful in the diagnosis of diffuse brain dysfunction, and occasionally their asymmetry can be of localizing value. In this section we consider only those reflexes that are easiest to elicit and evaluate. The subject has been reviewed recently by Paulson.[15]

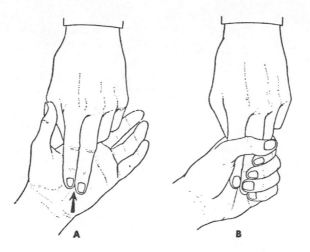

FIGURE 2-6. Grasp reflex. (A) Palmar stimulation; (B) grasp response. (From Paulson, G.W.,[15] with permission.)

Grasp Reflex

A grasp reflex is said to be present when a distally moving tactile stimulus to the palm results in grasping of the stimulating fingers or object (Fig. 2-6). The resulting grasp may be firm enough to entrap the stimulus, in which case release can be effected by a firm stroking movement on the back of the hand. At times it may be difficult to differentiate a true grasp reflex from a grasp secondary to habit or an attempt to cooperate. The grasp reflex has been linked to frontal lobe disease. A unilateral grasp reflex suggests contralateral cerebral disease.

Snout and Sucking Reflexes

These reflexes consist of a puckering or protrusion of the lips (secondary to contraction of the orbicularis oris) in response to a stimulus applied to the mouth area. To this may be added turning toward the stimulus, tongue movements, and even on occasion swallowing. The snout reflex is elicited by gently tapping the upper or lower lip (Fig. 2-7); and the sucking reflex, by a tactile stimulus (finger or tongue blade) applied to the same area. The reflexes normally are present in infancy and disappear with maturation, but they may reappear with diffuse cerebral dysfunction or bilateral corticobulbar disease.

Palmomental Reflex

This reflex consists of contraction of the mentalis muscle ipsilaterally

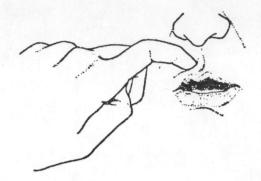

FIGURE 2-7. Snout reflex. Puckering of lips in response to gentle percussion in the oral region. (From Paulson, G.W.,[15] with permission.)

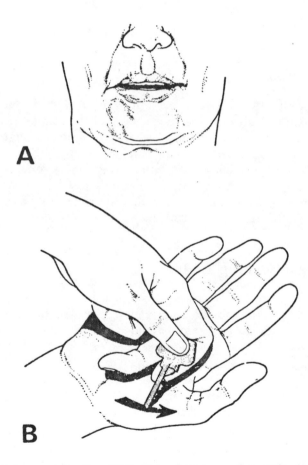

FIGURE 2-8. Palmomental reflex. (A) Ipsilateral response of mentalis muscle to (B) stimulation of thenar eminence. (From Paulson, G.W.,[15] with permission.)

following brisk stroking of the thenar eminence (Fig. 2-8). It, too, is usually present in infancy, becomes less significant with maturation, and frequently regains prominence in old age, especially with diffuse cerebral disease. Its emergence has been attributed to frontal lobe disease, but its localizing value is probably not so exact. A unilateral palmomental reflex may point to disease of the contralateral cerebral hemisphere.

Glabella Tap Reflex

Light tapping over the glabella (with the examiner's hand and percussing instrument held outside the field of vision so as not to elicit an avoidance response) normally evokes reflex blinking. In the normal subject, this disappears quickly with repetition, but in patients with a variety of cerebral diseases (most commonly involving both hemispheres or the basal ganglia), the blinking fails to disappear with repetitive stimulation (Fig. 2-9). A positive glabella tap response is characterized by this failure to wane on repetition.

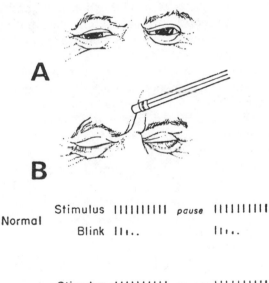

FIGURE 2-9. Glabella tap reflex. (A) Eyes at rest; (B) response to stimulus. Below are graphed normal and abnormal responses to repetitive stimuli. (From Paulson, G.W.,[15] with permission.)

Nuchocephalic Reflex

In 1975, Jenkyn and associates[11] described the nuchocephalic reflex, a previously undescribed primitive reflex present in infancy, inhibited in healthy adults, and present with diffuse cerebral dysfunction. The subject stands with eyes closed (to avoid visual fixation), and the examiner turns the shoulders briskly to either right or left. In the normal adult, the subject's head turns in the direction of the shoulder movement after a time lag of about one-half second. The reflex is said to be present if the subject's head holds its original position (necessitating bilateral reflex contraction of cervical musculature).

INTERPRETATION OF THE NEUROLOGIC EXAMINATION

The best of neurologic examinations is worth little if the psychiatrist cannot utilize the observations made. The practicing psychiatrist cannot be expected to perform and interpret the neurologic examination with the sophistication of the neurologist or neurosurgeon, but he or she should be able to uncover evidence of significant organic dysfunction, localize the probable site(s) of lesions when dysfunction is detected, identify the more common neurologic syndromes, and recognize those situations that merit referral for more extensive evaluation. Here only a few guidelines to interpretation can be suggested.

First, the physician must be constantly aware that a normal neurologic examination does not exclude the existence of significant neurologic disease. Some major disorders (such as epilepsy) may manifest no abnormalities on clinical examination. Others, by virtue of their localization in so-called silent areas of the brain (such as the frontal lobes) may be difficult to detect by the conventional examination. Still others, such as some of the diffuse cerebral degenerative processes, may fail to produce abnormal signs until the disease is far advanced. Thus the normal neurologic examination means *just* that the examination was normal, not that organicity has been excluded.

We turn now to some of the basic inferences that can be made when abnormalities are uncovered:

1. Neurologic abnormalities limited to one extremity or to a portion of one extremity are most likely due to spinal root or peripheral nerve disease.
2. Neurologic abnormalities limited to areas below a particular dermatome level with preservation of function above suggest spinal cord disease.
3. Crossed motor or sensory loss (one side of face and opposite side of body) or bilateral dysfunction of the cranial nerves and the extremities is likely the result of brain stem disease.

4. Dysfunction limited to one half of the body suggests disease involving one cerebral or cerebellar hemisphere. Cerebral hemisphere disease results in dysfunction of the contralateral half of the body; cerebellar hemisphere disease, in dysfunction of the ipsilateral half.

Other features help to localize dysfunction in the motor sphere. Figure 2-10 lists the motor and reflex findings characteristically associated with lesions at different levels of the neuromuscular apparatus. This table is a guide to help localize those lesions which impair motility, but the physician must remember that these changes are not invariably present with the diagnosed lesions, and that the changes may be mixed because the lesions involve more than a single level of neural function. Furthermore, such a simplified table does not include all the relevant details; for example, the distribution of weakness may be important, symmetrical proximal weakness being characteristic of primary muscle disease, symmetrical distal weakness of peripheral neuropathy.

Lesion of the sensory pathways usually can be localized with equal precision. The following are helpful but not invariable guidelines:

1. Sensory loss in a relatively well circumscribed area of the face, trunk, or an extremity is most likely due to spinal root or peripheral nerve disease.
2. Bilateral, essentially symmetrical sensory loss, greatest distally in the extremities (in a stocking-glove distribution), is usually the result of peripheral neuropathy. With peripheral neuropathy, the transition between areas of sensory loss and areas of normal sensation is usually gradual.

Lesions of:	Spontaneous Movements	Weakness	Atrophy	Fascicu-lations	Ataxia	Muscle Tone	Muscle Stretch Reflexes	Babinski Sign	Involuntary Movements
Cerebral Cortex and upper motor neuron	↓	+	O	O	O	↑	↑	+	O
Basal Ganglia	↓ ↓	O	O	O	O	↑	N	O	+
Cerebellum	N	O	O	O	+	↓	N	O	O
Lower Motor Neuron	N	+	+	+	O	↓	↓	O	O
Neuromuscular Junction	N	+	O	O	O	N	N	O	O
Muscle	N	+	+	O	O	↓	↓	O	O

N = normal   + = present   O = absent   ↑ = increased   ↓ = diminished

FIGURE 2-10. Neurologic abnormalities with lesions at different levels of the neuromuscular apparatus. The chart is merely a guide; individual variations are frequent.

3. Sensory loss (especially if complete) affecting an entire extremity or part of an extremity below a band-like level of abrupt transition is usually a manifestation of a conversion reaction.
4. Loss of sensation below a dermatome level with normal sensation above usually indicates spinal cord disease. With spinal cord lesions, the zone of transition may be narrow, but the change is not as abrupt as with most conversion reactions.
5. Crossed sensory loss (one side of the face and the opposite side of the body) is usually due to brain stem disease.
6. Sensory loss confined to one side of the body (cranium, trunk, and extremities) is probably due to a lesion of the contralateral hemisphere. When sensory loss is dense and extends exactly to the midline, the possibility of a conversion reaction should be entertained.
7. Unilateral sensory loss involving primarily the finer sensory modalities (two-point discrimination; object, weight, and texture recognition, and so forth) and largely sparing pain and touch suggests disease of the contralateral sensory cortex.

Interpretation of soft neurologic signs and primitive reflexes requires special care. None of these signs or reflexes found in isolation has predictable clinical consequences. Soft neurologic signs are of especial use in the evaluation of younger patients with learning problems, behavioral difficulties, and emotional disorders. The presence or absence of these signs can serve as a clue to the role neurologic dysfunction is playing in the patient's difficulties. Unfortunately, the absence of soft signs does not rule out organic involvement, nor does their presence predict an identifiable neuropathologic lesion. The presence of several soft signs does, however, suggest that neurologic dysfunction plays at least some role in the patient's disorder.

The demonstration of primitive reflexes is most useful at the other end of the age scale, in middle-aged and elderly subjects. Here, too, the presence of several of these primitive reflexes does not permit the prediction of an identifiable neuropathologic lesion, but it does strongly suggest that neurologic dysfunction is playing some role in the patient's neuropsychiatric dysfunction.

Jenkyn and coworkers[12] recently looked systematically for a number of soft signs and primitive reflexes in a group of patients with diffuse cerebral dysfunction. From the 32 signs and reflexes for which they searched, they identified the following as most useful in providing evidence of diffuse brain dysfunction: nuchocephalic reflex, glabella tap reflex, suck reflex, limitation in vertical gaze, defects in visual pursuit, lateral gaze impersistence, paratonic rigidity of both arms and both legs, and abnormal limb placement. Unfortunately, no single sign or reflex was present in every patient with diffuse brain disease and at the same time was never falsely positive in the absence of brain disease.

These are at best only rudimentary guidelines for using the neurologic examination. We have not, in this chapter, touched on how the psychiatrist uses the history and examination to diagnose specific neurologic diseases. Those disease states most frequently encountered by psychiatrists and most likely to be confused with functional psychiatric disorders are considered in detail in succeeding chapters.

REFERENCES

1. Akhtar, S., and Buckman, J.: The differential diagnosis of mutism. A review and report of three unusual cases. Dis. Nerv. Syst. 38:558, 1977.
2. Bender, M.B., Fink, M., and Green, M.: Patterns in perception on simultaneous tests of face and hand. Arch. Neurol. Psychiat. 66:355, 1951.
3. Benson, D.F.: Psychiatric aspects of aphasia. Brit. J. Psychiatry 123:555, 1973.
4. Benson, D.F.: Disorders of verbal expression, in Benson, D.F., and Blumer, D. (eds.): Psychiatric Aspects of Neurologic Disease. Grune and Stratton, New York, 1975.
5. Benson, D.F., and Geschwind, N.: The aphasias and related disturbances, in Baker, A.B., and Baker, L.H. (eds.): Clinical Neurology. Harper and Row, New York, 1976.
6. Benton, A.L., Van Allen, M.W., and Fogel, M.L.: Temporal orientation in cerebral disease. J. Nerv. Ment. Dis. 139:110, 1964.
7. Bickerstaff, E.R.: Neurological Examination in Clinical Practice, ed. 3. Blackwell Scientific, Oxford, 1973.
8. DeJong, R.N.: The Neurological Examination, ed. 3. Harper and Row, New York, 1967.
9. DeJong, R.N.: Case taking and the neurologic examination, in Baker, A.B., and Baker, L.H. (eds.): Clinical Neurology. Harper and Row, New York, 1977.
10. Gerson, S.N., Benson, D.F., and Frazier, S.H.: Diagnosis: Schizophrenia versus posterior aphasia. Am. J. Psychiatry 134:966, 1977.
11. Jenkyn, L.R., Walsh, D.D., Walsh, B.T., et al.: The nuchocephalic reflex. J. Neurol. Neurosurg. Psychiatry 38:561, 1975.
12. Jenkyn, L.R., Walsh, D.B., Culver, C.M., et al.: Clinical signs in diffuse cerebral dysfunction. J. Neurol. Neurosurg. Psychiatry 40:956, 1977.
13. Joynt, R.J., Benton, A.L., and Fogel, M.L.: Behavioral and pathological correlates of motor impersistance. Neurology 12:876, 1962.
14. Mayo Clinic, Rochester, Minn., Department of Neurology: Clinical Examinations in Neurology, ed. 4. W.B. Saunders Company, Philadelphia, 1976.
15. Paulson, G.W.: The neurological examination in dementia, in Wells, C.E. (ed.): Dementia, ed. 2. F.A. Davis Company, Philadelphia, 1977.
16. Paulson, G.W., and Gottlieb, G.: Developmental reflexes: The reappearance of foetal and neonatal reflexes in aged patients. Brain 91:37, 1968.
17. Post, F.: Dementia, depression, and pseudo-dementia, in Benson, D.F., and Blumer, D. (eds.): Psychiatric Aspects of Neurological Disease. Grune and Stratton, New York, 1975.
18. Rochford, J.M., Detre, T., Tucker, G.J., et al.: Neuropsychological impairments in functional psychiatric diseases. Arch. Gen. Psychiatry 22:114, 1970.

19. Rodin, E.A.: Impaired ocular pursuit movements. Diagnostic value. Arch. Neurol. 10:327, 1964.
20. Slater, E.: Diagnosis of "hysteria." Brit. Med. J. 1:1395, 1965.
21. Slater, E., and Glithero, E.: A follow-up of patients diagnosed as suffering from "hysteria." J. Psychosom. Res. 9:9, 1965.
22. Steegman, A.T.: Examination of the Nervous System: A Student's Guide, ed. 3. Year Book Medical Publishers, Chicago, 1970.
23. Strub, R.L., and Black, F.W.: The Mental Status Examination in Neurology. F.A. Davis Company, Philadelphia, 1977.
24. Warrington, E.: Constructional apraxia, in Vinken, P., and Bruyn, G. (eds.): Handbook of Clinical Neurology, Vol. 4. North-Holland Publishing Company, Amsterdam, 1969.
25. Weintraub, M.I.: Hysteria. A Clinical Guide to Diagnosis. Clinical Symposia (Ciba) 29:#6, 1977.
26. Wells, C.E.: Neurological Evaluation in General Practice. World-Wide Abstrs. Gen. Med. 9:#1, 8 and 9:#2,8, 1966.

CHAPTER 3

DELIRIUM

Lipowski[8] wrote that delirium was "the Cinderella of English-language psychiatry: taken for granted, ignored and not considered worthy of study." Although much has been published in the decade following the appearance of his paper, the statement otherwise remains accurate. Yet delirium, without question, is the organic brain syndrome most frequently encountered by psychiatrists, both in patients admitted to hospital psychiatric units and in patients seen for consultation on other services. Engel[3] estimated that 10 to 15 percent of all patients hospitalized on acute medical and surgical services manifested some degree of delirium, and if only the elderly are considered, the percentage doubtless is even higher. Its prevalence is possibly even greater on acute psychiatric services, but the exact incidence is unknown. Delirium is often overlooked, often misdiagnosed, and often not recorded among the discharge diagnoses, having only been a transient phase in a long and complex illness. Every psychiatrist needs a thorough understanding of delirium, for it is the psychiatrist to whom others turn when diagnostic uncertainty or problems in symptomatic management emerge.

The term delirium is derived from the Latin *de* (from or out of) plus *lira* (furrow or track); the delirious patient is thus "off the track" or "out of the rut." Even its derivation, therefore, implies a deviation from the individual's usual state. Delirium is also a common lay term, and to date it lacks a codified, widely accepted medical definition. Many synonyms thus have emerged—toxic psychosis,[2] metabolic encephalopathy, syndrome of cerebral insufficiency,[4] exogenous metabolic brain disease,[11] acute brain syndrome.[1] The latter has been the accepted diagnostic rubric for psychiatrists since 1968, but it appears likely that the classic term delirium will return to psychiatric nosology with the third edition of the *Diagnostic and Statistical Manual*. The common denominator for the condition referred to by all these terms is that it reflects, as Cohen[2] wrote, "some distortion of cerebral cellular metabolism," and that it

45

does not arise primarily within the brain but is a response of the brain to insult from without, whether that insult be metabolic, chemical, infectious, or traumatic.

Delirium is defined here as a symptom complex manifested by:

1. An acute or subacute onset
2. Marked clinical variability from patient to patient and from time to time in the same patient
3. Diffuse dysfunction of neural tissue including the cerebral hemispheres, the reticular activating system, and usually the autonomic nervous system
4. Essentially complete reversibility
5. The absence both of pathognomonic neuropathologic changes during the acute phase and of significant residual pathologic changes when early recognition has prompted effective treatment.

Delirium and dementia (discussed in Chap. 5) are the two common neuropsychiatric syndromes manifested by global cognitive impairment. In some ways these syndromes stand at opposite poles, but it must also be recognized that there is a continuum between them so that at times labeling a patient's disorder one or the other is more a matter of opinion than of medical certainty (see Table 1, Chap. 4) Also, it is not uncommon for delirium to result eventually in dementia or to be superimposed on dementia.

CLINICAL FEATURES

General

Delirium usually is acute or subacute in onset, i.e., it develops into a clinically recognizable syndrome over a period of several hours to several days. Less commonly, delirium can develop insidiously over a period of weeks, this being more likely when due to slowly developing endocrinopathies (e.g., hypothyroidism) or deficiency disorders (e.g., pernicious anemia).

Prodromata, such as daytime restlessness, insomnia, and vivid, frightening dreams or nightmares are not unusual, but their significance as the first symptoms of organic psychosis is usually appreciated only in retrospect. If the symptoms are observed and recognized as heralds of delirium, two maneuvers have been described that might confirm the diagnosis. The first is study of the visual images elicited by light pressure or gentle massage of the closed eyes. Ordinarily nondelirious patients report patterns of light and color upon the darkness, but with early delirium formed objects or even complex tableaux may be seen.[15,17] Another technique is to ask the patient to look carefully at a sheet of clean white paper or at a blank wall and to report what is seen.

Again, with early delirium vivid hallucinatory experiences are sometime reported in this situation.[17] Early diagnosis is important, not only for treatment of the delirium itself, but because psychologic disintegration may be a "sensitive indicator of something going wrong systemically,"[17] i.e., it may warn of deterioration in the patient's medical condition.

The clinical presentation of delirium is likely to be more dramatic when its cause is sudden in onset (the brain accommodates better to slowly changing than to rapidly changing conditions). Onset may be marked by the loss of some important mental capacity (e.g., loss of alertness or interest) or by the addition of something decidedly abnormal (e.g., hallucinations, panic). The former is usually referred to a quiet delirium, the latter, a loud or violent delirium. Quiet delirium is as easily overlooked by psychiatrists in the psychiatric hospital as by other specialists in the general hospital. Patients with loud delirium (i.e., patients whose behavior disturbs others) are those whom psychiatrists are usually asked to see in consultation or to admit to psychiatric inpatient services.

Delirium is marked by clinical variability, so much so that Wolff and Curran[19] many years ago suggested variability to be its hallmark. Delirium may be so mild that it is difficult to recognize or so severe that it is life threatening. Clinical differences are striking not only from patient to patient (Lipowski[8] notes that one encounters depressive, paranoid, schizophrenic, phobic, and hysteric clinical pictures "reactive to the underlying cognitive impairment"), but variability is often marked in the same patient. At one time apathy or depression may predominate, and, at another, agitation and assaultiveness. The clinical course is also often punctuated by brief periods of near lucidity.

Delirium may be especially difficult to recognize when superimposed on a pre-existing psychosis. In such instances, the psychiatrist's first impulse often is to attribute the change to a worsening of the underlying psychosis. In this case, antipsychotic medications may be increased and further worsen the delirium, and a search for other causes for the worsening may be neglected. Continued awareness of the possibility of delirium in the psychiatric patient population (especially in those receiving large amounts of medications) lessens the chance for such errors.

The symptoms and signs of delirium are almost predictably worse at night than during the day. Some patients indeed become delirious only at night, regaining their lucidity when daylight returns. Several factors contribute. Illusions and hallucinations may be facilitated by darkness itself. In addition, insomnia is often severe, and prolonged loss of sleep may itself cause delirium. Furthermore, nights are times when there is a relative paucity of sensory stimulation, and sensory deprivation too

47

may cause delirium. Still, a completely satisfactory explanation for this diurnal variation is lacking.

Disturbance of Consciousness

Some alteration in the level of consciousness is a *sine qua non* for the diagnosis of delirium. Rather than define consciousness, which is often at best a quasi-philosophical concept, we will describe what we mean by its disturbance. In delirium a change in the level of consciousness may be manifested by: (1) a reduction in *awareness* of self and surroundings or (2) a change in attentiveness (alertness, vigilance, arousal) to the self and surroundings. The delirious patient's awareness is always reduced; the delirious patient's vigilance may be either increased or decreased. Change in awareness varies from a slight loss of registration of details to stupor (wherein the patient becomes aware of the environment only with effort) to coma (see Chap. 4). Change in vigilance or arousal ranges from serious apathy to marked excitement and agitation. Even with marked arousal, however, awareness of self and environment is defective.

Disturbances of Perception

Perceptual defects, ubiquitous in delirium, are closely related to disorders of consciousness. Despite their frequency and severity, perceptual defects have not been extensively studied in delirium, perhaps because so many patients cannot cooperate for detailed evaluations. Nonetheless, impaired perception is easily detected clinically, and even the fairly attentive patient fails to "take in" significant details concerning self and situation.

DISORIENTATION

Some degree of disorientation is usually demonstrable in delirium. The delirious patient characteristically first becomes disoriented to time, losing track of the hours, confusing morning with afternoon, day with night, then jumbling days, dates, months, and years. The disorientation to time is not stable, however, for patients may place themselves in one year at one moment and in another only a few moments later. Disorientation to place usually follows with worsening. This spatial disorientation is usually of a sort typical for delirium, i.e., patients mistake the unfamiliar for the familiar. Thus patients misidentify the hospital room as the bedroom at home or an ambulance as their personal station wagon. The phenomenon of double orientation is also sometimes seen, that is the sense of being in two different places at the same time. Most delirious patients maintain perception of who they are despite disorientation in other spheres, although this too may be lost as the patient nears coma.

ILLUSIONS

Illusions (erroneous or misinterpreted sensory impressions) are common in organic brain disease and rare in functional psychiatric disorders. They may result from stimulation by any sensory modality, but visual and tactile illusions are most common. A curtain fluttering at the window is misperceived as an intruder; a sheet, as a coat or napkin; a bedpost, as a walking stick. Although common objects may be misidentified, there is a tendency to misperceive the unfamiliar for the familiar; for example, the arrival of a meal tray may cause the patient to believe the hospital room to be a familiar restaurant. In this situation, spatial disorientation and illusion cannot always be clearly differentiated. Misinterpretations may also serve as the basis for delusional beliefs. Wolff and Curran[19] gave several examples: "They are breaking me to pieces," (painful arthritis); "feet cut off" (painful feet in a post-typhoid delirium); "tongue cut off" (sore tongue in postoperative delirium).

Illusions are especially common when environmental factors make sensory discrimination difficult. Thus visual illusions are likely when the delirious patient is placed in semidarkness; auditory illusions occur where competing sounds are many. In such settings a clear distinction between hallucinations and illusions cannot always be made.

HALLUCINATIONS

Hallucinations (perceptions occurring without recognizably relevant sensory stimulation) are common in delirium. Again, any sensory modality can be involved, but visual hallucinations are most common. The form and content of the hallucinatory experiences vary widely, from vividly colored hallucinatory forms to complex figures. In some delirious patients, hallucinations can be precipitated merely by closing the eyes. Not uncommonly, visual hallucinations are devoid of personal implication, an unusual occurrence in functional psychiatric illnesses. Hallucinations of animals are especially frequent, by no means being limited to the deliria associated with alcoholic excess. Some patients hallucinate objects of ominous significance—hearses, hell, funerals, coffins, and mechanisms for execution. Hallucinations too are more common where discrimination of sensory stimuli is difficult.

Disturbances of Thinking

Thought processes are defective in delirium, and usually the examiner can demonstrate the dysfunction with little effort. The patient often appears uninterested and attention wanders. Concentration is poorly sustained, with frequent digressions from any set topic. At other times perseveration in thought and speech occurs, thus demonstrating a defective capacity for altering attention to focus on a new topic. Even with perseveration, however, thoughts are often fragmented and reasoning defective. The capacity for organized, purposive behavior is reduced, and behavior may be determined by a single consideration to the neglect of other important factors. Problem solving is defective, and the patient may be baffled and overwhelmed by new and unfamiliar materials. Thought processes are usually slowed, but pressure of thoughts may dominate in excited states.

DELUSIONS

Delusions (false beliefs elaborated by the individual to satisfy inner needs) are common; they often appear to be elaborated from misinterpretations (illusions). As a rule, delusional ideas in delirium are fleeting and poorly systematized, and patients usually can be convinced that their delusions are unfounded. At times, however, delusions of danger or persecution can be so intense that the patient flees or jumps from a window because of the delusional belief. Paranoid attitudes are common and may dominate the clinical picture.

MEMORY

Memory is impaired, varying from a slight uncertainty about recent events to severe loss with dense lacunae for both recent and remote events. There is impairment in registration, retention, and recall of memories, and testing usually demonstrates defects in immediate, recent, and remote memories. Patients are often unable to maintain proper temporal sequences for those memories which can be recalled. A type of confabulation may be seen in which a patient ties together several unrelated memories in a sequence unrelated to their proper temporal order.

Upon recovery, patients are often able to recall little of what happened in the course of their deliria. Registration of memories was defective, perhaps due to impaired attentiveness and awareness, and those memories which can be recalled are often fragmented and fuzzy. On the other hand, vivid hallucinations are sometimes recalled with considerable clarity, an observation suggesting that the memory defects result not so much from an interference with memory mechanisms per se as with impaired perceptual and attentive processes.

OTHER INTELLECTUAL FUNCTIONS

Impairment of all intellectual functions can usually be demonstrated in well established delirium. Defects in performance of virtually all the tests of general intellectual function described in Chapter 2 are likely.

Disturbances of Affect

Lability is perhaps the most conspicuous affectual disturbance in delirium. At times affect is blunted; at times, intensified. Depression, anxiety, fear, anger, elation, and suspiciousness have all been described, but seldom is one affect pervasive and lasting. Mood often reflects impaired perceptions, illusions, and delusions, and the lability is further evidence of the variability of these processes. Most patients experience deeply, if fleetingly, disturbed affect in the course of a delirium. Euphoria or anger may be so intense that controlling behavior is a major problem, and depression can be so severe that suicide is a danger.

Disturbances of Psychomotor Activity

Patients may show a decrease and/or an increase in psychomotor activity. A decrease evokes little concern, but an increase may cause significant clinical problems. Restlessness may be intense with the patient in constant motion—tossing, turning, squirming, kicking, rubbing, picking, or searching. Miming of stereotyped, familiar, or occupational activities occurs and may be perseverated again and again.

Disturbances of Motility

A fine-to-coarse, rapid, irregular tremor at 8 to 10 per second is common. This tremor, usually minimal at rest, is accentuated by reaching for or grasping an object and by trying to maintain a fixed posture. Isolated rapid, jerky movements of the head, extremities, and trunk may be seen, as may ataxia, dysarthria, and dysprosody.

Two specific abnormalities of motility—asterixis and multifocal myoclonus—require special consideration because of their relative specificity for delirium. Asterixis is elicited by asking the patient to maintain a position with the arms extended, wrists dorsiflexed, and fingers extended. Asterixis (any involuntary, irregular, asymmetric jerking movements which follow) varies in intensity from slight lateral movements of the fingers at the metacarpophalangeal joints to brisk palmar flexion movements of the fingers and hand. These movements cannot be prevented by the patient even with effort. Although asterixis most often is described as a feature of hepatic encephalopathy, it may occur in delirium of any etiology. Bilateral asterixis is virtually pathognomonic of delirium.

Multifocal myoclonus is an abnormal involuntary movement caused by quick, asymmetric, arrhythmic, but at times repetitive contractions of muscles or muscle groups and occurring at rest. Multifocal myoclonus may involve widespread body areas, but the muscles of the face and shoulders are usually most prominently involved. Multifocal myoclonus, too, is almost a pathognomonic sign of delirium. Posner[11] suggested that it occurs later and at a more severe stage of illness than does asterixis.

Only asterixis and multifocal myoclonus possess any degree of diagnostic specificity for delirium; *all* other signs and symptoms are nonspecific.

Autonomic Dysfunction

Autonomic dysfunction, frequently serious and widespread, may help differentiate delirium from other types of neuropsychiatric dysfunction. Almost any symptom or sign of autonomic dysfunction may be encountered—nausea, vomiting, diarrhea, constipation, incontinence, flushing, pallor, blood pressure aberrations, sweating, palpitations, tachycardia, and fever. At times these may be life threatening; for example, the hyperpyrexia of delirium tremens can lead to death. To some extent, these autonomic changes may result from changes in affect and behavior—anxiety, fear, agitation, excitement—but this does not explain their occurrence entirely.

Posner[11] pointed out that changes in autonomic activity are at times of diagnostic assistance. Loss of pupillary light reactions usually suggests a structural lesion, but there are three exceptions in delirium: glutethimide produces mid-position or slightly dilated fixed pupils; anticholinergic drugs, dilated fixed pupils; and severe anoxia, dilated fixed pupils.

Hypothermia in delirium suggests myxedema, hypoglycemia, or barbiturate intoxication. Hyperthermia without sweating suggests anticholinergic drug intoxication or infection. Hyperthermia with profuse sweating and tachycardia may occur in any agitated delirium, although perhaps most commonly with delirium tremens. Posner also emphasized the diagnostic value of hypoventilation and hyperventilation as indicators of specific metabolic derangements (and he provided a complex but useful table to direct the physician in this evaluation).

THE CAUSES OF DELIRIUM

Although the diagnosis of delirium can usually be established clinically, the clinical picture often gives little hint as to etiology. Rarely does a specific clinical observation (such as pupillary change or hypothermia) suggest a specific etiology. Recurrent deliria in the same person are closely alike, even when their causes differ.

Furthermore, delirium often is the result of more than a single cause.

In the delirious patients studied by Cohen,[2] he noted that it was usually possible "to discern a major and several lesser reasons for the disturbance." We emphasize as well the frequency with which many factors converge to precipitate delirium. It is not unusual to find one or more predisposing factors plus one or more acute factors joining to tip the scales toward delirium.

Predisposing Factors

Although every person can become delirious under certain circumstances, there is a wide variation in human susceptibility. Some people fail to develop delirium even with considerable provocation, whereas others develop delirium repeatedly with minimal provocation. The possibility of a constitutionally determined proclivity to delirium has been suggested, but evidence for hereditary predisposition is lacking.

Delirium is said to be more common at the extreme ages of life, but the evidence of childhood susceptibility is scant. Geriatric patients unquestionably carry an increased predisposition to delirium. Two other groups also have increased susceptibility to delirium: (1) persons addicted to drugs or alcohol or with a history of addiction and (2) persons with brain damage of any type, sustained at any age. In addition, patients with chronic cardiac, pulmonary, hepatic, or renal dysfunction, even if insufficient to cause delirium itself, carry an increased vulnerability.

Individuals with certain personality characteristics, especially the paranoid personality, are described as being unusually vulnerable to delirium, but there is little solid supporting evidence. The same is true for the suggestion that patients with psychiatric dysfunction or with a history of psychiatric disease are unusually susceptible. Intense psychologic reactions—anxiety and fear in particular—are reported to predispose to delirium, and there is some evidence that patients most fearful of medical and surgical procedures have the highest incidence of complicating delirium.

Environmental factors, such as darkness and sensory deprivation, predispose and may at times be sufficient cause for delirium.

Precipitating Factors

Factors which can precipitate delirium seem endless in number, and articles describing hitherto unreported causes appear regularly in the medical literature. Table 3-1 lists in schematic form those that are most important, i.e., causes that must be considered in most patients. More detailed lists of causes can be found elsewhere.

Pathophysiology

Delirium is believed to occur whenever any acute or subacute disorder diffusely impairs cellular function of the nervous system. This results most frequently from extracranial factors, but exactly the same neuropsychiatric picture emerges whenever intracranial disease processes abruptly impair brain function diffusely (i.e., epilepsy and post-ictal states, subarachnoid hemorrhage, meningitis, encephalitis). In the latter disorders, the pathophysiologic basis for the clinical disruption is easily proved. In the primary extracranial disorders, however, what evidence do we have to verify the organic nature of the brain dysfunction? Evidence comes largely from studies in two areas—the electroencephalogram (EEG) and cerebral blood flow.

The EEG is a sensitive device for demonstrating changed brain function in delirium.[13] In every EEG study in which EEGs have been obtained in the same patient in both the delirious and the nondelirious states, EEG changes have been demonstrated in the midst of the delirium.[12] Most often there is a slowing of the dominant EEG rhythm during delirium, but in agitated deliria a shift in the opposite direction often occurs. This shift in dominant rhythm is ample evidence of altered brain function during delirium.

Supporting evidence comes also from cerebral blood flow and oxygen utilization studies (recently summarized by Sokoloff[16]). Neither oxygen nor glucose is stored to any significant extent in the brain, so that cerebral oxygen utilization is a good measure of brain metabolism. Cerebral oxygen utilization (uptake) is significantly diminished in delirium, the decrease being roughly proportional to the severity of the clinical manifestations. Cerebral blood flow may or may not decline in delirium, the changes in this function not always paralleling changes in oxygen uptake.

PATHOLOGY

By definition, delirium is marked by an absence of pathognomonic neuropathologic changes during the acute phase. This does not mean that gross and microscopic study of the brains of patients dying during delirium uniformly reveal no pathologic changes, but it does mean that the changes sometimes observed are nonspecific (i.e., they point to no specific etiology) and that they are largely reversible in patients who survive.

The pathologic changes described are usually distributed bilaterally, symmetrically, and diffusely in the cerebral hemispheres. Cerebral swelling, with widening of the perivascular and perineuronal spaces, is common. In addition, swelling of the neurons of the cerebral cortex and hippocampus, some dissolution of the Nissl granules, and generalized pallor may be seen on microscopic examination. These changes are largely reversible. With severe and prolonged delirium, more ominous pathologic changes appear, many of which are probably not reversible (and thus merge into the diagnosis of dementia).

DIAGNOSIS

Delirium should be suspected in every patient with recent onset of a change in level of consciousness, thinking, or behavior—and especially in those with no history of prior psychiatric dysfunction. Once suspected, careful attention to details of the history and mental status examination usually allows the diagnosis to be accepted or rejected.

The history often must be obtained from relatives and friends. In a disorder of such protean etiology, a detailed and meticulous history is essential—all bases must be touched. Aside from the history, the mental status examination is the chief diagnostic instrument. In delirium, the physician must structure the mental status evaluation so that it is brief but provides the basic information required. Most delirious patients have reduced attentiveness, concentrate poorly, and tire easily, so that prolonged questioning is impossible.

In suspected delirium the neurologic examination may reveal altered psychomotor activity and motility, both of which help to establish the correct diagnosis. More importantly, the neurologic examination in delirium reveals no focal neurologic defects. Signs of focal dysfunction raise the spectre of a localized organic lesion and dispel the likelihood of delirium (unless the delirium is in a patient with a pre-existing focal lesion). The general physical examination is vital, because it may uncover one or more of the many systemic diseases that cause delirium.

Differential Diagnosis

Delirium must be differentiated from schizophrenia, hysteria, and dementia. The history and mental status examination usually permit accurate differentiation among these.

SCHIZOPHRENIA

In schizophrenia, there is usually no alternation in the level of consciousness. Furthermore, even if the schizophrenic patient has marked disorganization of thought processes, both awareness of and attentiveness to the examiner are often preserved. The schizophrenic is usually not disoriented, but if so, the disorientation is likely to be bizarre and remote. The delirious patient usually mistakes the unusual for the usual; the schizophrenic, the usual for the unusual. The disoriented delirious patient, with diminished awareness, often appears to have no inkling that the physician is skeptical of proferred responses; the disoriented schizophrenic often appears not to expect the physician to believe, nor does the schizophrenic care. Intensive but fleeting affects are characteristic of delirium, whereas schizophrenic affect is likely to be aloof, distant, and flat. When paranoid delusions occur, the delirious patient often perceives a communal danger, but the schizophrenic is likely to perceive the harm as directed toward the patient alone. The schizophrenic patient personalizes; the delirious patient generalizes. Hallucinations are more often visual than auditory in delirium; the reverse holds for schizophrenia. When cooperation can be obtained, the schizophrenic usually shows little or no evidence of memory loss or general cognitive impairment, the characteristic changes of delirium. The delirious patient almost always has insomnia, with nocturnal exacerbation of symptoms and sometime improvement in the morning hours, but the schizophrenic often sleeps soundly, the symptoms persisting in full force on awaking. Asterixis and multifocal myoclonus are not features of schizophrenia.

HYSTERIA

In the hysterical neuroses, orientation is usually preserved. When disorientation occurs, the hysterical patient is frequently disoriented to person—a rarity except in the most advanced stages of delirium. Cognitive functions too are usually maintained in hysteria, but when diminished cognition occurs, it is often out of keeping with the patient's obvious alertness and responsiveness. Hallucinations are rare in hysteria, but when present they often have an air of both the theatrical and the naive. Again, asterixis and multifocal myoclonus are not features of hysteria.

DEMENTIA

Dementia usually is slow and insidious in onset, so that it is difficult to date the beginning with certainty; the onset of delirium can usually be fixed rather exactly. Changes in the level of consciousness are rare in dementia until it is far advanced, whereas they are a feature of delirium from the outset. Hallucinations are seldom the prominent feature in dementia that they are in delirium, and they seldom appear early. Autonomic dysfunction is rare in dementia in contrast to its prominence in delirium. Asterixis is not seen in dementia, and although multifocal myoclonus may be seen, it usually appears only in far advanced disease. Dementing diseases predispose patients to the development of delirium, and thus delirium is often encountered in patients with pre-existing dementia.

Other disorders occasionally present differential diagnostic problems.

An acute manic episode may mimic an agitated delirium, but the absence of changes in consciousness, the preserveration of memory and other cognitive functions (when these can be adequately evaluated), and pervasiveness of the euphoria rule against the diagnosis of delirium. Transient global amnesia (see Chap. 14) presents an even rarer problem. In this disorder, limitation of the dysfunction to the amnestic sphere rules out the diagnosis of delirium.

The clinical picture will occasionally be so unclear that the physician cannot be certain whether or not the patient is delirious. Longer observation often clears the diagnostic confusion, but the patient can be so sick that expectant observation is ill-advised. In such rare instances, immediate electroencephalography may be helpful. If the EEG reveals diffuse slow activity in the theta and delta range without focal defects, this is strong evidence for the diagnosis of delirium. EEGs whose dominant activity lies within the usual range of normal and those with predominantly low-voltage fast records may occur in delirium, so that these records neither confirm nor rule out delirium. Thus the characteristic diffusely slow EEG can help make the diagnosis, but a normal or fast record does not rule it out. This subject has recently been reviewed.[12] The EEG also occasionally may demonstrate unsuspected subclinical status epilepticus,[18] a rare cause of delirium but an important diagnosis because of the specificity of its treatment.

PATIENT MANAGEMENT

No foolproof recipe for the management of delirium is available, nor will one be forthcoming. Much depends on the setting in which the delirium is seen. Delirium coming on during the course of inpatient psychiatric treatment calls for a different response from delirium in the postoperative state, which in turn demands a different approach from delirium seen in the emergency room, especially if in the latter no history is available. Once delirium is diagnosed on the basis of its clinical features, attention must be given to three tasks: (1) identification of the precipitating cause or causes; (2) their specific treatment; (3) emergency treatment and symptomatic treatment for nonspecific signs and symptoms of the delirium. Even though these three tasks may be dealt with separately in discussion, in practice the patient's condition may require that they be carried out simultaneously.

Although identifying the cause of delirium is important, it is not unusual for a delirium to come and go without its cause being found; conversely, so many possible causes may be identified that it is impossible to define the exact role of any single factor. In the neatest of situations, the history or physical examination provides clues for specific disorders. Sometimes, however, the best of histories offers no clue or no history is available, so that the search for cause begins without helpful leads. Drugs and their withdrawal are always suspected, but determination of blood and urine levels takes time and may not be available when the initial diagnostic formulation must be made.

Although the primary central nervous system disorders listed in Table 3-1 not infrequently cause delirium, their incidence is not high

TABLE 3-1. Causes of delirium

I. Primary Brain Dysfunction
  1. Epilepsy and post-ictal states
  2. Trauma (especially concussion)
  3. Infections
    a. Meningitis
    b. Encephalitis
  4. Subarachnoid hemorrhage
II. Secondary Brain Dysfunction
  1. Drugs (ingestion and withdrawal) and poisons
    a. Sedatives (including alcohol)
    b. Tranquilizers
    c. Other drugs
      Insulin
      Salicylates
      Steroids
      Cardiac glycosides
      Anticonvulsants
    d. Poisons
      Carbon monoxide
      Heavy metals
  2. Endocrine dysfunction (hypofunction or hyperfunction)
    a. Pituitary
    b. Thyroid
    c. Parathyroid
    d. Pancreas
    e. Adrenal
  3. Diseases of nonendocrine organs
    a. Liver (hepatic encephalopathy)
    b. Kidney and urinary tract
      Uremic encephalopathy
      Electrolyte imbalance
    c. Lung
      Carbon dioxide narcosis
      Hypoxia
    d. Cardiovascular system
      Cardiac failure
      Cardiac arrhythmias (especially cardiac arrest)
      Hypotension
    e. Deficiency diseases
      Thiamine deficiency (Wernicke's encephalopathy)
      Vitamin B_{12} or folate deficiency
    f. Miscellaneous disease states
      Infections with fever and sepsis
        (not intracranial infections)
      Electrolyte imbalance of whatever cause
      Postoperative states

when all cases of delirium are considered. Nevertheless, their recognition is important. When a history of trauma or seizures is obtained, or when focal neurologic signs or nuchal rigidity are observed, the possibility of brain disease per se should be pursued immediately with appropriate diagnostic studies. These are not necessary in every delirious patient, however, especially not in those in whom other causes seem more likely.

Since delirium is most often secondary to disease processes located outside the brain, the physician looks first for the most common offenders. Among the endocrine disorders, diabetes is a frequent cause, and delirium may result from either hypoglycemia or hyperglycemia. Delirium is common with fever and sepsis. Hepatic disease sufficient to cause hepatic encephalopathy is usually accompanied by jaundice, spider angiomata, hepatomegaly, fetor hepaticus, or ascites, but these rarely can be absent even with severely deranged liver function. Urinary tract disease causes delirium secondary to uremia, infection with fever and sepsis, and disorders of electrolytes and osmolality. Examination of the chest should reveal signs of pulmonary dysfunction severe enough to cause delirium. Cardiovascular function must be assessed, for changes in blood pressure, cardiac output, and cardiac rhythm may result in delirium.

Usually disease of the organ systems discussed above will be evident clinically, but occasionally this is not the case, and more information will be needed. When the etiology of the delirium is not established and diagnostic clues are sparse, initial laboratory procedures usually should include the following: electrolytes, blood urea nitrogen, liver function tests, arterial PO_2 and PCO_2, blood and urine for determination of sedative and tranquilizer levels, urinalysis, and electrocardiogram.

Because an almost limitless number of disorders exist, the treatment of specific disorders which cause delirium is obviously beyond the scope of this chapter.

Emergency Treatment

Delirium is often a neuropsychiatric emergency. In such an emergency, the physician may not have enough time for a complete and systematic evaluation but may have to deal with life-threatening problems first, deferring detailed examinations until after these have been dealt with. Conditions that immediately threaten life or permanent brain damage and hence must be treated at once include: hypoglycemia, diabetic ketosis and hyperosmolality, hypoxia and anoxia, hyperthermia, and Wernicke's encephalopathy (see Chap. 8).

HYPOGLYCEMIA

Hypoglycemia is usually the first thought when a known diabetic under treatment develops delirium. In other situations, this possibility may not be so apparent. Because severe, prolonged hypoglycemia causes irreversible brain damage, every delirious patient in whom an etiology is uncertain should be treated to correct possible hypoglycemia. After blood has been drawn for immediate glucose determination and a urine specimen checked for ketosis, the patient should be given 50 ml of 50 percent dextrose solution intravenously. This may not bring about immediate improvement if the patient has been hypoglycemic for some time, but it prevents further cerebral damage pending definitive diagnostic studies.

DIABETIC KETOSIS AND NONKETOTIC HYPEROSMOLALITY

In the recognized diabetic, delirium should be suspected to result also from diabetic ketosis or nonketotic hyperosmolality. On occasion diabetes may even present with one of these complications manifested chiefly by delirium. Hyperpnea, the odor of acetone on the breath, dehydration, and hypotension point to a diagnosis of diabetic ketosis, and hyperglycemia, glucosuria, and ketosuria establish the diagnosis. Marked hyperglycemia and glucosuria in the absence of ketosuria make the diagnosis of nonketotic hyperosmolality likely. Insulin plus intravenous saline are the emergency treatments of choice in either condition, with further fluid replacement being determined by monitoring of blood electrolytes and acid-base balance.

HYPOXIA AND ANOXIA

Because sustained hypoxia or anoxia results in permanent brain damage, their immediate recognition and correction are essential. Cerebral hypoxia may result from decreased oxygen content of circulating blood (due to pulmonary disease, anemia, carbon monoxide poisoning) or from interference with blood flow to the brain (due to cardiac arrest, cardiac arrhythmias, myocardial infarction, hypotension). These possibilities must be investigated quickly and remedial measures taken at once to prevent further damage.

HYPERTHERMIA

Hyperthermia may cause death in delirious patients. With severe hyperthermia, quick corrective measures using alcohol sponges, ice packs, and fans may be life saving.

Nonspecific and Symptomatic Treatment

In this section we deal with general principles of treatment, i.e., measures aimed not at treating the cause of the delirium but measures applicable regardless of the cause. Three areas will be considered: (1) management of the environment, (2) medical support, and (3) medications for symptomatic relief.

ENVIRONMENT

The delirious patient functions best in a quiet, simple, and orderly setting. Excessive and conflicting sensory stimuli aggravate cerebral disorganization as, at the other end of the spectrum, does sensory deprivation. The physician should structure the best possible environment to reduce stress on the delirious patient. This usually consists of a private, simply furnished, well lighted room which is quiet but not absolutely silent. Because darkness increases dysfunction, the room should be kept well lighted at all times. Constant attendance is needed, especially when the delirium is severe; the fewer the number of different attendants, the better. Two or three trusted relatives or friends and two or three nursing personnel over a 24-hour period are most desirable. Family and friends should be thoroughly instructed about the nature of the disorder and the role they should play in attendance. The attendants' task is largely one of reassurance and prevention of injury. The attendant must orient the patient repeatedly to time, place, and situation and reassure the patient again and again of his safety. Medical and nursing personnel should be clearly identified, by dress if possible, and they should introduce themselves to the patient at each encounter and state why they are there and what they are doing. Diagnostic and therapeutic procedures should be explained thoroughly each time to lessen the patient's apprehension and obtain cooperation. Attendants constantly must be wary to protect the patient from self-injury. Physical restraints should be used sparingly, but at times their use is not only unavoidable but therapeutic.

MEDICAL SUPPORT

Supportive medical care is often important, even when it is not directed against the cause of the delirium. Incessant hyperactivity leads to fever and exhaustion. Insomnia is often severe and debilitating. Inadequate food and fluid intake results in severe dehydration, electrolyte imbalance, or vascular collapse. Close monitoring of the patient's medical status is a necessity.

MEDICATIONS

Not every patient with delirium requires medications for symptomatic relief. Medications may even be contraindicated, especially in patients with significant depression in their level of consciousness. Medications are most useful in reducing feelings of fear, anxiety, irritability, anger, and panic, and in controlling aggressiveness, restlessness, hyperactivity, and insomnia. They do little specifically to improve disorientation, memory loss, cognitive dysfunction, or perceptual abnormalities, although these functions may improve with reduction in fear and anxiety. Because virtually all medications that reduce fear, anxiety, and anger have a potential for further decreasing the level of awareness (and thus increasing the severity of delirium), their use demands caution and careful monitoring of response.

For years hypnotic drugs were mainstays in symptomatic treatment for delirium; they are little used today. Tranquilizers are now the medications of choice, and rarely is there cause to use the older sedatives and hypnotics. The benzodiazepines, especially chlordiazepoxide and diazepam, have been used extensively and have been proved reliable.[7] They produce minimal depression in consciousness, minimal cardiovascular and respiratory effects, and are anticonvulsants, an added feature of value when delirium results from withdrawal of alcohol and drugs. Given in adequate amounts, they rarely fail to achieve effective control. Antipsychotic agents (major tranquilizers) also have been employed in delirium, but for several reasons they are still not considered by many authorities to be drugs of first choice in most instances. They may produce considerable depression in the level of consciousness, cardiovascular side effects are not uncommon, and some are said to be epileptogenic. Heller,[6] on the other hand, recommended the use of phenothiazines or haloperidol in all deliria except for the withdrawal syndromes.

For moderate anxiety and restlessness in the young or middle-aged adult, 25 to 50 mg chlordiazepoxide (Librium), 5 to 10 mg diazepam (Valium), or 15 to 30 mg oxazepam (Serax) might be given initially. For more severe anxiety and agitation, initial doses of 50 to 100 mg chlordiazepoxide, 10 to 20 mg diazepam, or 30 to 60 mg oxazepam might be chosen. Parenteral administration may be necessary initially in the uncooperative patient, but quicker, higher, and more sustained blood levels of chlordiazepoxide and diazepam are achieved through the oral route than intramuscularly[14] (oxazepam is not available in a parenteral preparation). For the assaultive or panicked patient, 50 mg chlordiazepoxide or 10 mg diazepam given slowly intravenously may be required initially. In elderly patients and those with known cerebral damage, an initial dose of 10 mg chlordiazepoxide, 2 mg diazepam, or 15 mg oxazepam might be chosen. Repeated doses of the chosen medication are usually given every one to two hours until adequate control of the clinical symptoms is achieved. Each of these medications has a relatively long half-life, so that the physician must remember that accumulation of drugs and active metabolites is a danger with repeated administration. Haloperidol (Haldol), in doses of 2 to 5 mg intramuscularly every hour for several hours, has been reported to effect quick control of the deliria due to acute alcohol withdrawal.[9,10] Its effectiveness for longer periods and over a broader range of deliria has not been reported.

Therapy with these medications aims to control target symptoms and promote light sleep but to prevent excessive sedation. As Greenblatt and Shader[5] stated: "When therapy is inadequate, symptoms rage on, while overdosage produces obtundation, coma, and respiratory depression." Titrating the dosage to achieve a mid-position between these extremes is often difficult.

OUTCOME

Lipowski[8] outlined four possible outcomes of delirium: (1) full restitution to premorbid state; (2) transition to dementia or another organic mental disorder; (3) transition to a nonorganic mental disorder (schizophrenic, paranoid, affective, hysteric); (4) death (due to brain dysfunction or to primary extracranial disease processes). Although delirium is invariably transient (unless death occurs), its lifting does not therefore invariably result in full return to the premorbid state, even though this is undoubtedly the most common course. The longer delirium goes unrecognized or persists despite treatment, the greater is the likelihood of permanent brain damage; and, thus, even though the delirium eventually lifts, the patient will suffer residual organic impairment. Transition to a nonorganic mental disorder is rare and suggests that the disorder was present but unrecognized before the delirium.

CONCLUSIONS

Delirium is the syndrome of organic brain dysfunction probably most frequently encountered by the psychiatrist. If this is kept in mind, the diagnosis of delirium on clinical examination is usually not difficult, and treatment is usually effective, quick, and gratifying to both the physician and the patient.

REFERENCES

1. American Psychiatric Association: Diagnostic and Statistical Manual of Mental Disorders, ed. 2. American Psychiatric Association, Washington, D.C., 1968.
2. Cohen, S.: The toxic psychoses and allied states. Am. J. Med. 15:813, 1953.
3. Engel, G.L.: Delirium, in Freedman, A.M., and Kaplan, H.I. (eds.): Comprehensive Textbook of Psychiatry, ed. 1. Williams and Wilkins Company, Baltimore, 1967, pp. 711-716.

4. Engel, G.L., and Romano, J.: Delirium, a syndrome of cerebral insuffi- ciency. J. Chron. Dis. 9:260, 1959.
5. Greenblatt, D.J., and Shader, R.I.: Treatment of the alcohol withdrawal syndrome, *in* Shader, R.I. (ed.): Manual of Psychiatric Therapeutics. Little, Brown and Company, Boston, 1975, pp. 211-236.
6. Heller, S.S.: The organic patient and medical problems, *in* Glick, R.A., Meyerson, A.T., Robbins, E., et al. (eds.): Psychiatric Emergencies. Grune and Stratton, New York, 1976, pp. 135-146.
7. Kaim, S.C., Klett, C.J., and Rothfeld, B.: Treatment of the acute alcohol withdrawal state: A comparison of four drugs. Am. J. Psychiatry 125:1640, 1969.
8. Lipowski, Z.J.: Delirium, clouding of consciousness and confusion. J. Nerv. Ment. Dis. 145:227, 1967.
9. Palestine, M.L.: Drug treatment of the alcohol withdrawal syndrome with delirium tremens. A comparison of haloperidol with mesoridazine and hy- droxyzine. Q.J. Stud. Alcohol, 34: 185, 1973.
10. Palestine, M.L., and Alatorre, E.: Control of acute alcoholic withdrawal symptoms: A comparative study of haloperidol and chlordiazepoxide. Curr. Ther. Res. 20:289, 1976.
11. Posner, J.B.: Delirium and exogenous metabolic brain disease, *in* Beeson, P.B., and McDermott, W. (eds.): Cecil-Loeb Textbook of Medicine, 14th ed., Vol. I. W.B. Saunders Company, Philadelphia, 1975, pp. 544-552.
12. Pro, J.D., and Wells, C.E.: The use of the electroencephalogram in the diagnosis of delirium. Dis. Nerv. Syst. 38:804, 1977.
13. Romano, J., and Engel, G.L.: Delirium. I. Electroencephalographic data. Arch. Neurol. Psychiat. 51:356, 1944.
14. Shader, R.I., and Greenblatt, D.J.: Clinical implications of benzodiazepine pharmacokinetics. Am. J. Psychiatry 134:652, 1977.
15. Small, S.M.: Psychological and psychiatric problems in aged and high-risk surgical patients, *in* Siege, J.H., and Chodoff, P.D. (eds.): The Aged and High Risk Surgical Patient. Grune and Stratton, New York, 1976, pp. 307-328.
16. Sokoloff, L.: Circulation and energy metabolism of the brain, *in* Albers, R.W., Siegel, G.J., Katzman, R., et al. (eds.): Basic Neurochemistry. Little, Brown and Company, Boston, 1972, pp. 299-325.
17. Titchener, J.L., Zwerling, I., Gottschalk, L., et al.: Psychosis in surgical patients. Surg. Gynecol. Obstet. 102:59, 1956.
18. Wells, C.E.: Transient ictal psychosis. Arch. Gen. Psychiatry 32:1201, 1975.
19. Wolff, H.G., and Curran, D.: Nature of delirium and allied states. Arch. Neurol. Psychiatry 33:1175, 1935.

CHAPTER 4

COMA AND STUPOR

If asked to see a patient in coma or stupor, the psychiatrist can be certain that the patient poses a diagnostic or therapeutic problem. Usually coma and stupor are dealt with by other physicians—specialists in family or emergency medicine, internists, neurologists, neurosurgeons—so that psychiatric consultation is likely to be requested only if the primary physician concludes or strongly suspects that the state is not organic in nature.

In addition, in the psychiatrist's own practice, a few patients with identified emotional or mental disorders will become stuporous or comatose and create diagnostic and therapeutic problems. Is the changed state of consciousness a rare but well described manifestation of the primary psychiatric process? Does it result from a toxic reaction to prescribed medications taken in usual amounts or from an overdose of medications (whether suicidal in intent or not)? Is it the consequence of organic brain disease, either previously present but unrecognized or newly superimposed on the primary psychiatric disorder?

Whatever the situation in which the psychiatrist encounters stupor or coma, the same question must be asked and answered: Does the patient's reduced level of responsiveness result from organic or from psychologic causes? To rely on other specialists to answer this question is to be vulnerable to errors of both commission and omission. Certain nonorganic stupors (depressive stupor, for example) are familiar only to psychiatrists and thus may appear "organic" to the nonpsychiatrist who has never encountered them before. Conversely, certain organic states (petit mal status, for example) may appear "functional" to the physician unfamiliar with them. The psychiatrist must develop expertise in making these differentiations in order to identify which patients should be treated by standard psychiatric techniques and which by other specialists using other techniques.

TERMINOLOGY

In this chapter we deal with clinical disorders in which patients *appear* to experience primarily some alteration in their level of consciousness. We define consciousness operationally (as did Plum[7]) as the process of awareness both of the environment and of the self. Awareness is, of course, a subjective state, not precisely measurable by external monitoring devices. Practically speaking, awareness can be assessed only by evaluating the patient's capacity to interact meaningfully with the environment and with persons in the environment. Thus, as in so much of psychologic medicine, we seek to assess an inner experience (awareness of self and environment) through behavioral observation and measurement. We infer defective awareness on the basis of behavioral change. Most of the time this inference is justified.

In Chapter 3 (Delirium) we discuss the most common clinical disorder in which deviation from normal levels of alertness and awareness is a necessary and prominent feature. In delirium, however, despite an altered level of awareness, responsiveness to the environment is usually preserved to a significant degree. In this chapter, we consider more profound deviations from normal levels of awareness, as manifested by strikingly reduced responsiveness to the environment, and we deal with both the organic and the nonorganic or psychogenic states in which these changes occur.

Coma was defined by Plum and Posner[9] as a state of "unarousable unresponsiveness." In coma, the patient is completely unresponsive to internal as well as to external stimulation. Such patients are unlikely to be seen by psychiatrists, who are more likely to see patients in a state best referred to as stupor. Plum[7] defined stupor as "a state wherein subjects respond when vigorously stimulated, but immediately sink back again as soon as external stimuli are withdrawn." Joyston-Bechal[6] described stupor as a "basic triad consisting of akinesis, mutism, and relative preservation of consciousness," going on to observe that the assumption that consciousness was relatively preserved might be "based on the presence of eye movements which appear purposeful rather than random." These patients cannot then be aroused fully but retain some responsiveness to physical stimulation (e.g., wincing or slight withdrawal to pain, pupillary constriction to light, preservation of some response to pharyngeal stimulation). Over the years many terms—clouding of consciousness, confusional states, light coma, semi-coma—have been used to describe the stuporous states. Teasdale and associates[11] recently highlighted the unreliability which attends use of these terms in describing the stuporous patient. They pointed out that only precise description of the patient's behavior and responsiveness to external stimulation permits consistent and reliable monitoring of the clinical course.

66

CLASSIFICATION AND CAUSES

Plum and Posner[9] classified the causes of stupor and coma as follows: (1) supratentorial lesions; (2) subtentorial lesions; (3) metabolic disorders; (4) psychiatric disorders. Supratentorial lesions accounted for the altered states of consciousness in about 18 percent of Plum and Posner's cases. Only rarely, however, did the stupor or coma result solely because of the dysfunction of the supratentorial tissue itself. Most of the time, supratentorial lesions produced coma when either edema (surrounding an infarct or a mass) or a tumor caused downward pressure resulting in damage to the diencephalic or midbrain structures that normally arouse and activate the cerebrum. Primary subtentorial lesions comprised a little over 13 percent of their series. These lesions (mainly infarctions but including a few tumors, hemorrhages, and abscesses also) resulted in coma either due to destruction of the paramedian midbrain-pontine reticular formation by the lesion itself or due to compression of the reticular substance by extrinsic lesions.

Over two thirds of Plum and Posner's cases were due to metabolic disorders, by which they meant any disorder that resulted in failure of neuronal metabolism. These might be intrinsic diseases of neuron or neuroglia (e.g., Alzheimer disease), which they termed primary metabolic encephalopathy, or extrinsic disorders that resulted in diffuse neuronal dysfunction, which they termed secondary metabolic encephalopathy. The vast majority of their cases were due to secondary metabolic encephalopathy. These would be equivalent to severe and far advanced delirium, as discussed in Chapter 3.

In only 4 of Plum and Posner's original 386 patients was the coma or stupor due to psychiatric disorders. Studies from psychiatric facilities suggest that psychogenic coma and stupor may occur more frequently than these figures would indicate, but perhaps such cases are not seen often on busy medical emergency services which were the sources of Plum and Posner's clinical material.

COMA

Coma is usually life threatening, and the neurologic examination usually gives evidence that brain function is severely compromised organically. Neurologic abnormalities are rarely out of keeping with the depression of consciousness in the comatose patient. Thus, as noted above, Plum and Posner[9] made a diagnosis of psychogenic unresponsiveness in only four of their patients, although the diagnosis had been suspected at first in several others. In their opinion, coma on a psychogenic basis "sustained for more than a few minutes is uncommon."

The diagnosis of psychogenic coma rests not only on the absence of pathologic neurologic signs but also on the presence of other consistently observable findings. In psychogenic coma, blood pressure and pulse are usually normal, but there may be tachycardia. Respirations are normal or rapid in rate; neither Cheyne-Stokes respirations nor sustained tachypnea is observed. Pupils respond normally to light. These patients usually lie immobile with their eyes closed. Often there is resistance to opening the eyes (usually absent when coma is on an organic basis). Obviously, such resistance demonstrates a high level of sensitivity to and responsiveness to external stimulation. When the eyelids are held open, the eyes do not manifest the slowly roving side-to-side movements often observed in organic disease, and when the eyelids are released, they do not close slowly and gradually as is usual in organic states. Fisher[3] suggested that these roving eye movements and gradual eyelid closure are not mimicked in psychogenic obtundations, but it is difficult to believe that anything observed in organic diseases of the nervous system will not at some time also be observed in psychogenic states.

There is usually diminished resistance to passive movement of the extremities, but in psychogenic states, if an extremity is moved brusquely, momentary initial resistance may be felt. A grimace or some element of withdrawal may be observed in response to tickling the nostril with a wisp of cotton or stimulation of the extremities with the point of a pin. Corneal and gag reflexes are characteristically preserved—but they are occasionally missing in psychogenic coma. The patient usually swallows spontaneously, and pooling of secretions is not often a significant problem. Muscle stretch reflexes are usually normal but may be hypoactive, and superficial abdominal and cremasteric reflexes are brisk and symmetrical. The plantar responses are ordinarily downgoing, but they too may rarely be absent. The picture presented is that of a patient unaware of the environment, unarousable, akinetic, and limp, but a patient otherwise without evidence of medical or neurologic dysfunction.

Except when there is compelling evidence to the contrary, a diagnosis of psychogenic coma or stupor should not be made in the absence of any of the following: (1) a normal neurologic examination (except for impaired responsiveness to both verbal and mechanical stimulation); (2) normal oculocephalic responses; (3) normal oculovestibular (caloric) reflexes; and (4) a normal electroencephalogram.

Oculocephalic and Oculovestibular Reflexes

Plum and Posner[9] emphasized the usefulness of the oculocephalic (doll's-head-eye phenomenon) and the oculovestibular (caloric) reflexes in the clinical evaluation of comatose and stuporous patients. The oculocephalic reflex is sought by rotating the head briskly from side-to-side (or by briskly flexing and extending it) while holding the eyes open. A positive response, i.e., a positive oculocephalic reflex, consists of conjugate movement of the eyes in the direction opposite to that in which the head is moved (e.g., conjugate deviation of the eyes toward the right when the head is rotated toward the left). In normal, awake subjects, oculocephalic responses are inconsistent, probably dependent in large part on the degree of visual fixation. The oculocephalic reflex becomes more consistently present in awake patients with bifrontal or diffuse hemispheric dysfunction and in those with stupor and coma of organic origin.

Caloric stimulation is performed by irrigating the external auditory canal with cold water. The canal must be free of cerumen and the head elevated 30° from the horizontal. The tip of a small catheter is placed near the tympanic membrane and, using a large syringe, ice water is slowly pushed through the catheter to irrigate the membrane. Irrigation is stopped as soon as nystagmus or deviation of the eyes occurs (or after 200 ml of cold water has been introduced if there is no response). The normal response to caloric stimulation is the appearance of nystagmus with the slow component toward and the fast component away from the irrigated ear. The nystagmus is regular and rhythmic, lasting up to two or three minutes, with little excursion of the eyes away from the midline.

In psychogenic coma, the oculocephalic response is inconsistent (as it normally is), and the response to caloric stimulation is normal as well. A normal response to caloric stimulation must be demonstrated before the diagnosis of psychogenic coma can be firmly established. Such a response to caloric stimulation does not occur in coma of organic origin. We agree with the admonition of Strub and Black[10]: "Do not diagnose psychogenic unresponsiveness too hastily; the misdiagnosis of a true coma as hysteria is far more serious than the reverse."

Electroencephalography

In patients whose clinical findings are inconclusive, the electroencephalogram may be diagnostic. A normal electroencephalogram is incompatible with a diagnosis of coma due to organic causes (or, at the very least, exceptions to this rule are so rare that they demand considerable deliberation and questioning). On the other hand, an abnormal EEG does not prove that the coma is necessarily secondary to the usual organic causes, for abnormal EEGs are not unusual in schizophrenic catatonias (although admittedly an organic origin for these has not been disproven).

Psychopathology

Perhaps because of its relative rarity, the psychopathology underlying psychogenic comas has not been thoroughly studied. It appears that psychogenic comas are most likely secondary to catatonic schizophrenia or to hysteria (being perhaps a form of hysterical psychosis), but more facts are needed.

STUPOR

For the psychiatrist, stupor is a more difficult differential diagnostic problem than coma. It is much more difficult to differentiate psychogenic from organic stupor than to make the same differentiation in coma, because the features that separate psychogenic from organic stupor are not nearly so clear-cut. Let us look first at the characteristics of the psychogenic stupors and examine those features that help to separate them from the more frequent organic stupors.

Psychogenic Stupor

In psychogenic stupor, a variable awareness of the environment appears to be preserved. At one end of the spectrum, patients lie most of the time with their eyes closed and rouse only briefly with verbal or physical stimulation. At the other end of the spectrum, the eyes are kept open most of the time, looking about with what appears to be some degree of interest. Patients may lie motionless, show occasional postural movements, or even move on command and assist in eating or cleansing. Painful stimulation results in no visible response in some and in vigorous movements to push the stimulus away in others. Some patients with psychogenic stupor remain completely mute, while others occasionally utter monosyllables or even short phrases. They may swallow their secretions, food, and liquid placed in their mouths or require pharyngeal suctioning and tube feeding. Both urinary and fecal incontinence may occur.

In catatonic stupor, other features often blur the distinction between psychogenic and organic stupors even further. Low grade fever is common, as is tachycardia, tachypnea, and sweating. The pupils are often dilated, but they respond to light, and even anisocoria has been described. Grimaces and choreiform jerks of the extremities are common. The arms and legs are often held rigid and resist movement, but at other times a waxy flexibility (also seen in organic stupors) is present.

Thus many features commonly seen in organic disease are often present in psychogenic stupor, and other differential diagnostic observations helpful in coma may be of little value in stupor. Although abnormalities of oculocephalic and oculovestibular reflexes always suggest organic disease, normal reflexes are compatible with organic stupors. Furthermore, an EEG which is within normal limits is compatible with organic stupor, and an abnormal EEG is compatible with catatonic stupor.

Differential Diagnosis

In differentiating organic from psychogenic stupor, the psychiatrist must turn to other observations for diagnostic assistance; unfortunately none of these is pathognomonic. The history is often helpful. Stupor coming on in the course of severe depression, schizophrenia, or hysterical neurosis (especially if the patient is not taking large amounts of psychotropic medications) is more likely to be psychogenic in origin than stupor appearing with no history of psychiatric dysfunction. On the other hand, catatonic stupor may appear suddenly in young persons without previously recognized emotional problems, and organically caused stupor may occur in patients with longstanding psychiatric disease.

A careful and detailed neurologic examination is perhaps the single most important diagnostic aid. It is rare for patients with organic stupor to have *no* neurologic abnormalities demonstrable by careful and detailed examination. The abnormalities are not necessarily conspicuous, but even minor deviations from normal make a complete neurologic investigation mandatory before making a diagnosis of psychogenic stupor.

Another helpful though not diagnostic sign is mutism (see Chap. 2). In the absence of gross neurologic deficits, is most commonly a sign of psychiatric, not of neurologic, dysfunction.[1] In a patient who can be aroused and who has a normal neurologic examination, mutism points strongly toward a psychogenic state. Except in the acute phase, complete muteness is an uncommon manifestation of aphasia; it rarely occurs in neurologic disease otherwise except in far advanced degenerative disorders.

The sodium amytal interview may be helpful.[12] Intravenous barbiturate usually deepens organic stupor. On the other hand, it often results in temporary improvement in psychogenic stupors, bringing about increased verbalization and cooperation. Obviously barbiturates must be administered with caution in possible organic stupors, but the diagnostic information to be gained may well make the slight risk acceptable. Failure to improve with intravenous amytal, however, by no means rules out psychogenic stupor.

It is often said that organic and psychogenic stupors can be distinguished in retrospect by whether or not the patient recalls what transpired during the stuporous period. In Joyston-Bechal's excellent study[6] of 100 stuporous patients, however, on follow-up evaluation only a minority with proved psychogenic stupors had total recall of the stuporous period.

The identification of those stupors which are psychogenic from the totality of stuporous states is not easy. Many times, no certain distinction between psychogenic and organic stupor can be made immediately, and only detailed study and close, continued observation permits an exact diagnosis.

Psychopathology

The identification of psychogenic stupor does not provide the psychiatrist with a diagnosis of the underlying psychopathology. Although catatonic schizophrenic stupor has received most attention, Joyston-Bechal[6] found that stupor due to depressive illness occurred almost as often as that due to schizophrenia. Stupor was seen also with significant frequency in a group of patients with hysterical features plus depression, a group labeled "mixed neurotic" by Joyston-Bechal. In his series, no clinical feature of the stupor itself permitted diagnosis of the underlying psychiatric disorder.

We have emphasized thus far that only with careful study is the diagnosis of psychogenic stupor made with reasonable certainty. To reach this conclusion, there obviously must have been something about the patient's state to raise this suspicion, because by far most stupors are organic in origin. Usually psychogenic stupor is suspected when there is incongruence between the apparent level of awareness and responsiveness to speech and/or to the manipulations of the neurologic examination. Thus, when the patient appears unaware of the environment but maintains normal responsiveness on neurologic examination, or when the patient appears alert but responds poorly to verbal questions or commands, a psychologic basis for the stupor should at least be suspected.

We turn next to some specific neurologic disorders in which this incongruence occurs, disorders which the inexperienced physician might label incorrectly as psychogenic on the basis of this incongruence.

SPECIFIC NEUROLOGIC DISORDERS MANIFESTED BY STUPOR

Akinetic Mutism

We use the term akinetic mutism to refer to a variety of states that result from lesions involving the reticulocortical pathways between the upper midbrain and the cortex, with or without associated cortical lesions. Despite the terminology, these patients are not necessarily either completely akinetic or totally mute. Other terms used to describe these syndromes, depending on the specific clinical manifestations and the specific location of lesions, are *coma vigil,* the apallic state, and persistent vegetative state.[5] Plum's description of the state as one of "permanent mindlessness" is especially apt.[8] Earlier in their illness, most of these patients have been comatose, from which they have "awakened" to this state of permanent mindlessness. These syndromes result from virtually any neuropathologic alteration involving the appropriate neural structures, but most commonly are due to infarction or trauma.

The clinical feature that sets these syndromes apart from others is the incongruence between the patient's severe and persistent hypokinesis and mutism and the appearance of awareness of the environment. This appearance of awareness varies considerably. Some patients lie with their eyes open most of the time, blinking normally, eyes roving conjugately about the room, at times fixing on objects or persons, even occasionally following moving objects. Others keep their eyes closed most of the time but can be aroused, by verbal or physical stimulation, to present the semblance of awareness just described. Despite this semblance of awareness, however, it is impossible to establish meaningful communication with these patients. Some appear to go through repeated cycles of waking and sleeping; others maintain a stance of persistent vigilance (*coma vigil*).

Accompanying this often eerie and uncanny appearance of awareness is some degree of persistent mutism and akinesis. These, too, vary in degree. Some patients never emit a sound, whereas others upon stimulation may grunt, moan, or even utter single words or brief phrases. Some remain persistently motionless except for eye blinks, conjugate eye movements, and respirations, whereas others upon stimulation make some purposeful movements of the extremities.

Neurologic examination is usually strikingly abnormal—snout reflex, grasp reflexes, spasticity, hyperactive muscle stretch reflexes, absent superficial abdominal reflexes, Babinski signs. In a few patients, however, neurologic examination is virtually normal, with only minor and uncertain deviations demonstrable. In these patients, the lesions are limited largely to the reticular pathways. It is in such instances that diagnostic errors are especially likely. Because of these particular patients with akinetic mutism, the psychiatrist cannot afford to dismiss even trivial evidence of neurologic dysfunction in patients with stupor.

The Locked-In Syndrome

The locked-in syndrome, a term coined by Plum and Posner,[9] results when a neurologic lesion, usually hemorrhage or infarction, completely interrupts corticobulbar and corticospinal pathways at the level of the upper pons. This results in preservation of cortical and midbrain function but loss of motor activity except for vertical eye movements and respirations. The important point is that these patients apparently retain full awareness of their environment, but their only avenue of response is blinking of the eyelids and vertical movement of the eyes. Using eyeblinks and eye movements as signs, communication can be established with the patient, so that at least minimal emotional and physical needs can be met. Otherwise the patient is totally "locked-in." Neurologic abnormalities are usually prominent, so that the disorder is unlikely to be confused with psychogenic coma except possibly in the acute phase, before the full gamut of abnormal neurologic signs has developed.

Kleine-Levin Syndrome[2,4]

The Kleine-Levin syndrome is characterized by recurrent bouts of hypersomnolence and hyperphagia, usually lasting for periods of several days to several weeks. It most often occurs in teenaged males, and it may be associated with a characteristic EEG abnormality (persistent high amplitude diffuse 2 to 3 Hz slow activity) during the periodic attacks. The cause of the disorder is unknown, and there is no specific treatment, but it tends to remit with time.

Patients with the Kleine-Levin syndrome can be awakened (sometimes with considerable effort) and will respond appropriately for brief periods, but if left alone, they sleep most of the day and night, awaking only to gorge themselves on food and to attend to toilet needs. They are often irritable on being awakened. Many psychiatric and neurologic symptoms and behavioral changes have been described during the attacks. The episodes remit spontaneously, and often only a partial memory of what transpired during the attack remains. Patients are usually described as normal neurologically and psychiatrically between episodes. There is in these subjects *no* incongruence between appearance and responsiveness which would suggest psychogenic stupor, but the bizarreness of the symptoms and behavior might suggest an hysterical disorder to the physician not familiar with the syndrome. The diagnosis rests on clinical observations and does not depend on the demonstration of EEG abnormalities.

SUMMARY

Psychiatrists sometimes are asked to see patients with stupor and coma for evaluation and treatment, usually because some lack of fit between the patients' apparent level of awareness and their responsiveness to stimulation suggests a psychogenic etiology. Psychiatrists should be wary of accepting the diagnostic conclusions of referring physicians and should refine their own diagnostic skills so that costly diagnostic and therapeutic errors are avoided.

REFERENCES

1. Akhtar, S., and Buckman, J.: The differential diagnosis of mutism. A review and a report of three unusual cases. Dis. Nerv. Syst. 38:558, 1977.
2. Critchley, M.: Periodic hypersomnia and megaphagia in adolescent males. Brain 85:627, 1962.
3. Fisher, C.M.: The neurological examination of the comatose patient. Acta Neurol. Scand. 45: Suppl. 36, 1969.
4. Gilbert, G.J.: Periodic hypersomnia and bulimia: The Kleine-Levin Syndrome. Neurology 14:844, 1964.
5. Jennett, B., and Plum, F.: Persistent vegetative state after brain damage. A syndrome in search of a name. Lancet 1:734, 1972.
6. Joyston-Bechal, M.P.: The clinical features and outcome of stupor. Br. J. Psychiatry 112:967, 1966.
7. Plum, F.: Introduction, and The pathogenesis of stupor and coma, in Beeson, P.B., and McDermott, W. (eds.): Textbook of Medicine, ed. 14. W.B. Saunders Company, Philadelphia, 1975, pp. 540-544.
8. Plum, F.: Personal communication, 1978.
9. Plum, F., and Posner, J.B.: The Diagnosis of Stupor and Coma, ed. 3. F.A. Davis Company, Philadelphia, 1980.
10. Strub, R.L., and Black, F.W.: The Mental Status Examination in Neurology. F.A. Davis Company, Philadelphia, 1977.
11. Teasdale, G., Knill-Jones, R., and Van der Sande, J.: Observer variability in assessing impaired consciousness and coma. J. Neurol. Neurosurg. Psychiatry 41:603, 1978.
12. Ward, N.G., Rowlett, D.B., and Burke, P.: Sodium amylobarbitone in the differential diagnosis of confusion. Am. J. Psychiatry 135:75, 1978.

CHAPTER 5

DEMENTIA

Although delirium is the organic brain syndrome encountered with greatest frequency, the possibility of dementia probably presents the psychiatrist with more differential diagnostic problems. Functional psychiatric disorders can mimic delirium, but they rarely mimic it very accurately. On the other hand, functional disorders often mimic dementia, and sometimes very well, so that differentiating dementia from pseudodementia is often challenging. The psychiatrist's job does not end, however, with the recognition of dementia. Recognition is just the beginning, and beyond lie the tasks of identifying its cause, treating the cause if possible, and ministering to the patient's needs as manifested by cognitive, affectual, and behavioral dysfunction.

Dementia is derived from the Latin *de* (from or out of) plus *ment* or *mens* (mind) plus *ia* (pathologic consideration). Taking into account its derivation alone, dementia would appear to refer to very nonspecific mentative changes; edition 25 of *Dorland's Illustrated Medical Dictionary* defines it as "a general designation for mental deterioration." However, dementia has come to have a specific meaning in contemporary medical usage, i.e., in medicine today, dementia refers only to the clinical syndrome that results from loss of brain function due to diffuse organic brain disease. Chronic brain syndrome is the most common synonym for dementia, a synonym which likely will be replaced by the classic term "dementia" in the third edition of the APA's *Diagnostic and Statistical Manual*.

Dementia is defined here as a clinical syndrome usually characterized by: (1) an insidious onset, chronicity, and progressivity; (2) brain dysfunction limited predominantly to the cerebral hemispheres; (3) pathologic changes in affected cerebral tissue demonstrable by both light and electron microscopy; and (4) ultimate irreversibility. This definition of dementia cannot, however, be stated without qualifications.[24] The onset in some dementias may be abrupt, as with those following cerebral trauma or anoxia. Nor are all dementias progressive, for example, the dementia following trauma or anoxia may be stable or even recede with the passage of time. In some dementias, e.g., Creutzfeldt-Jakob disease, dysfunction also may extend far beyond the cerebral hemispheres, and in others pathologic changes are not invariably present, at least early in the course. Thus, in early dementia due to hypothyroidism, the brain may appear normal structurally. Changes would, however, ultimately appear in this condition were the disease to go untreated. The same disorder remains reversible for some period, although again ultimately a point of no return is reached. These potentially reversible dementias, which Roth[19] has called "secondary dementias," are of especial diagnostic importance because of the possibility of restitution of function.

Dementia and delirium are contrasted in Table 5-1. It should be recognized that there is a continuum for each of these features between dementia and delirium, so that not every patient has every feature of one or the other syndromes.

Dementia also must be distinguished from mental retardation and from the changes of normal aging. Mental retardation refers to a stable condition, of multiple etiologies, usually present from the neonatal period, in which patients have reduced capacity for learning and for cognitive tasks in general. There is little reason for mental retardation to be confused with dementia clinically. Brain functions normally change with aging, so that in the elderly there is often mild loss of memory for recent events, slowed performance of set tasks, slowed acquisition of new knowledge, and unwillingness to take chances in situations of uncertainty. Serious impairment of mentative capacities with old age, however, always suggests significant brain damage and should never be accepted as normal.

TABLE 5-1. Features differentiating dementia from delirium

Dementia	Delirium
Chronic	Acute
Dysfunction largely confined to cerebral hemispheres	Widespread neural dysfunction
Characteristic pathologic changes	Pathologic changes absent or nonspecific
Irreversible	Reversible
Little variability in individual patient	Marked variability in individual patient
Single etiology	Multifactorial etiology

CLINICAL PRESENTATION

Defects in orientation, memory, intellectual functions, judgment, and affectivity are usually highlighted in descriptions of dementia. They are indeed the features that define chronic brain syndrome in the APA's *Diagnostic and Statistical Manual*.[1] These features often dominate the clinical picture, and they are universally prominent in the advanced stages. They are, however, often inconspicuous early in the course of the dementing process when diagnosis is likely to be a problem. Because dementia is usually a progressive process, the clinical picture is not fixed but changes and evolves with increasing loss of cerebral tissue. The clinical features are best understood by grouping the manifestations into the early, middle, and late phases of the disorder.

The Early Phase

The early symptoms are likely to be vague or to suggest more a functional psychiatric disorder than an organic brain disease. Somatic complaints are often prominent, and pain, weakness, anorexia, insomnia, constipation, bloating, dizziness, and a host of similar symptoms may prompt the patient to seek medical attention. The symptoms often fail to suggest any specific disease or to fit any recognizable syndrome. Depression and anxiety are often troublesome and sometimes pervasive, but lability of affect and mood swings are also common. Liston[14] has stressed the prominence of depressive symptoms early, and he showed that the affective symptoms may so capture the physician's attention that recognition of the underlying dementia is delayed.

The patient with early dementia often complains of irritability, and lowered frustration tolerance is noted by the patient and family. New situations, of a sort that would have been dealt with easily before, may prove baffling. Memory impairment is usually present to some degree, but it may not be a complaint. Many, perhaps most, patients appear to lack awareness of and concern for the defects in memory, while in those who do complain of forgetfulness, memory loss is more directly related to the severity of the accompanying depression than to the severity of the amnesia.[7]

Characteristic of this stage is the patient who struggles too hard to accomplish previously easy tasks; who expresses too much satisfaction from trivial accomplishments; who makes excessive use of lists, schedules, and notes; who neglects to return to a subject as promised; who is inappropriately revealing; who feigns indifference to the substance of a question, saying that the sons or daughters or spouse keep up with that sort of thing. There is diminished drive, diminished creativity, and diminished capacity for achieving satisfaction, often manifested by a constriction of interests, excessive concern about a few matters, and a general withdrawal from usual activities.

The manifestations of this early phase are commonly insidious and often so nonspecific that their significance is recognized only in retrospect, when overt signs of dementia have thrust the diagnosis upon the family and physician. Often long periods go by between the onset of symptoms and the seeking of medical assistance, an unfortunate delay for those with disorders amenable to specific treatment.

The Middle Phase

In this phase, the classic manifestations of organic brain disease, as enumerated in the *Diagnostic and Statistical Manual of Mental Disorders*[1] are apparent:
1. Impairment of orientation
2. Impairment of memory
3. Impairment of judgment
4. Impairment of all intellectual functions, such as comprehension, calculations, knowledge, learning, etc.
5. Lability and shallowness of mood.

Whereas earlier the patient may have presented as a diagnostic problem, in this phase the diagnosis is usually obvious; only the etiology remains in doubt.

As in delirium, orientation is usually lost first for time, later for place, and much later, if ever, for person. Recent memory usually suffers most, but remote memories disappear as well with progression of the disease, and the ability to organize memories into their proper temporal sequence disintegrates. Judgment fails, and patients may be so oblivious to their plight that reasoned judgment is impossible. All intellectual functions are impaired. Patients comprehend poorly what they see, hear, and read, and cannot assimilate their experiences. Their stores of information are both depleted and jumbled, and ability to learn new material is severely impaired. Calculations are faulty, and errors go unrecognized. Concentration span is severely limited. There is usually a progressive diminution of any preceding depression and anxiety, with progressive flattening of affect, though irritability and outbursts of anger or crying may persist.

During this phase personality change may be prominent. In some, this takes the form of an accentuation of previous personality characteristics, with excessive reliance upon a few premorbid defense mechanisms and coping devices. In others, atypical behavior emerges, much to the chagrin of family and friends. Personal dress and cleanliness may be ignored; concern for others often disappears. The drive for achievement withers, and failures are overlooked or go unrecognized. Hallucinations, illusions, and delusions may appear.

During the early phase of dementia, the neurologic examination usually remains normal. During the middle phase, signs of neurologic dysfunction often make their appearance, especially the emergence of so-called primitive reflexes as described in Chapter 2. These neurologic signs, most characteristic of diffuse brain disease, may not appear, however, until late in the disease, or not at all. Their appearance seems to depend more on the extent of brain damage and the speed of progression than upon other factors.[16]

The Late Phase

As damage progresses, apathy dominates, and the human substance of the personality is lost. Whereas earlier evidence of mentative incapacity dominated the clinical picture, in the terminal stage neurologic impairment predominates. Walking and other purposive movements are affected, and the patient becomes progressively confined to wheelchair and bed. Talking and swallowing are impaired. Contractures of the extremities follow, as do urinary and fecal incontinence. Depression of consciousness now supervenes, progressing usually to stupor or coma before death.

The early clinical manifestations are mostly in the sphere of psychologic dysfunction. In this phase, dementia may be easily confused with functional psychiatric disorders, and there is danger that the organic nature of the process will be overlooked. In the middle phase, the mentative signs of organic brain disease are blatant and unmistakable, but some functional psychiatric disorders (pseudodementias) mimic organic disease well, and there is danger here that the functional process will be overlooked. In the last phase, neurologic dysfunction predominates, and the danger of diagnostic error is nil.

In discussing the clinical characteristics of dementia, it is important to note that certain clinical manifestations of organic brain lesions are not characteristic of dementia. Specifically, the mentative changes due to focal cerebral lesions usually differ from those due to diffuse cerebral disease (i.e., dementia). With focal lesions, specific circumscribed mental functions are often impaired, sometime severely and in isolation. With diffuse disease, multiple mental functions are usually impaired, and often to about the same extent. For example, the aphasic patient may at first appear severely demented, but recognition of the aphasic defect may explain the entire clinical picture and point to a left hemispheric defect. Conversely, the presence of dense aphasia with sparing of other mentative functions is incompatible with diffuse cerebral disease.

CAUSES

The syndrome of dementia is usually diagnosed on clinical grounds (at times supplemented by ancillary diagnostic tests), but, as in delirium, the clinical picture often does not suggest a specific etiology. The clinical manifestations of dementia depend more on the extent and distribution of the cerebral lesions than on their specific pathology. The recognition of dementia must lead to a systematic consideration of possible etiologies. Table 5-2 lists the most common causes of dementia, with particular emphasis on those calling for specific therapeutic intervention. The reader is referred to the chapter by Haase[5] for a detailed treatment of these individual disorders.

The diffuse parenchymatous disorders have been relatively neglected

TABLE 5-2. Disorders causing dementia

PRIMARY CENTRAL NERVOUS SYSTEM DYSFUNCTION

Diffuse parenchymatous diseases of the central nervous system
    Alzheimer disease (presenile or senile form)
    Pick disease
    Parkinson disease*
    Huntington disease*
Trauma
    Open and closed head injuries*
    Subdural hematoma*
Brain tumors (primary or metastatic)*
Vascular disorders
    Atherosclerosis
    Multiple cerebral emboli*
    Prolonged sustained hypertension*
Normal pressure hydrocephalus*
Infections
    Postmeningitis or encephalitis
    Creutzfeldt-Jakob disease
    Syphilis*
    Cryptococcal meningitis*

SECONDARY CENTRAL NERVOUS SYSTEM DYSFUNCTION

Metabolic disorders
    Myxedema*
    Hypoglycemia*
    Chronic liver or renal failure*
    Hypoxia or anoxia*
Deficiency diseases
    Wernicke-Korsakoff syndrome*
    Vitamin B_{12} or folate deficiency*
Toxins and drugs
    Chronic alcohol abuse*
    Chronic abuse of sedatives or tranquilizers*
---

*Disorders calling for therapeutic intervention.

until recent years, but they are listed here first because Alzheimer disease is the single most frequent specific cause of dementia. Katzman and Karasu[10] estimated Alzheimer disease in its senile form to be the fourth or fifth most common cause of death in the United States. In the past most dementia, even if insidious in onset, has been ascribed to arteriosclerotic cerebral vascular disease. This was especially the case in elderly patients with cardiac or peripheral vascular disease, even though the correlation is known to be poor between peripheral vascular sclerosis and cerebral vascular sclerosis.

Cerebral vascular disease certainly may cause dementia, but Tomlinson, Blessed, and Roth[22] found that in elderly patients with typical dementia syndromes atherosclerosis alone accounted for only 18 percent of the cases and contributed significantly in another 18 percent. The senile form of Alzheimer disease, however, alone accounted for the dementia in 50 percent and played some part in another 18 percent. Four clinical series have also emphasized the central role of Alzheimer disease in the genesis of dementia.[4,9,15,21] On the other hand, when vascular disease is the cause, the clinical presentation usually differs from that of the diffuse dementing disorders.[24,26] Hachinski and coworkers[6] emphasized the usefulness of clinical features (such as abrupt onset, stepwise deterioration, fluctuating course, history or presence of hypertension, history of "strokes," focal neurologic symptoms, and focal neurologic signs) in distinguishing dementia due to vascular disease from that due to diffuse parenchymatous disease.

Appreciation of the importance of the parenchymatous degenerations has renewed interest in them, so that disorders such as Alzheimer disease, Pick disease, and Creutzfeldt-Jakob disease are now being studied with epidemiologic, biochemical, genetic, virologic, and immunologic methods.

PATHOLOGY

The cellular pathology of dementia depends, of course, upon the underlying disease; this large topic lies outside the scope of this book. It is important, however, to relate the neuropathologic alterations to the clinical manifestations, a topic basic to any understanding of dementia which recently has been reviewed elsewhere.[23]

Briefly stated, there is now data which directly relates the extent and severity of neuropathologic change to the severity of psychologic and social dysfunction. Specifically, severity of symptoms has been directly related to the mass of tissue loss,[2,12,30] the density of senile plaques and neurofibrillary tangles found in diseased brains,[18,22,23] and the mass of ischemic softening in affected brains.[22,23] Furthermore, in studies of the elderly, neuropathologic changes in the demented elderly have been found to be significantly greater than the changes in the nondemented elderly population.[23]

It is, therefore, axiomatic that a direct relationship exists between the severity of clinical dysfunction in dementia and the severity of neuropathologic damage.

DIAGNOSIS

Diagnosis depends on the history, mental status examination, and neurologic examination, sometime supplemented by ancillary testing procedures. The history, especially in the early phase, is apt to be unclear. During this time the patient's complaints are most likely to be considered functional in origin, and therefore the patient is likely to be referred for psychiatric evaluation. The history may confuse the physician further, because denial is often excessive and the truth does not easily emerge. Often only a history provided by family or friend can clarify matters. Unfortunately, all too often the family also denies the evidence for dementia, as when a highly intelligent husband recently explained that his totally disoriented wife "never did keep up with the days."

Even without specific symptoms of dementia, the physician should suspect it if the patient presents with:
1. Multiple somatic complaints fitting into no discernible pattern of physical disease, especially if this pattern of behavior is unusual for the person.
2. A variety of psychologic symptoms which fit into no specific functional diagnosis, especially in the patient with no prior psychiatric dysfunction of significance.
3. A story that appears muddled to the interrogator even after persistent and detailed questioning.
4. The development of delirium upon what appears to be slight provocation, thereby suggesting a lowered threshold to delirium due to underlying brain disease.

When the patient's complaints focus on emotional distress, the psychiatrist must avoid two specific diagnostic pitfalls; first, the tendency to consider all mental dysfunction in the young as functional; and second, the converse tendency to consider all mental dysfunction in the elderly as organic. Stated differently, there is a constant danger of failing to recognize organic cerebral syndromes in the young; there is a constant danger of failing to recognize functional disorders in the elderly.

The mental status examination described in Chapter 2 need not be detailed again here. We emphasize that the mental status must be consistently evaluated so that dementia is not overlooked. Paulson[16] wrote that "the *single* most valuable diagnostic clue to disorders such as Alzheimer's disease is the relative preservation of the neurologic state and the social graces in the presence of disintegrated memory and intellectual deterioration." He also noted that these patients use their defense mechanisms and cultural and educational background "to conceal the deficit with a pleasant smile and facile excuse offered to gloss over obvious errors as if they never existed."

A thorough mental status examination does not always prove diagnostic. Although deficits are uncovered, question may remain as to whether they are due to functional or to organic factors.

The physician then turns to the neurologic examination which may prove helpful by demonstrating either signs pointing toward a focal brain defect or signs (especially the emergence of primitive reflexes) suggesting diffuse disease.

By use of the history, mental status examination, and neurologic examination, the psychiatrist should be able to reach one of the following conclusions:

1. The patient has a functional disorder.
2. The patient has organic brain dysfunction due to a focal lesion.
3. The patient *may have* dementia, and if so it is probably due to diffuse cerebral disease.
4. The patient *has* dementia, most likely due to diffuse cerebral disease.

Patients in the first two categories usually cause the psychiatrist no further diagnostic problems. In the first group, the psychiatrist proceeds with treatment as though the question of dementia had not arisen. In the second, if the nature of the focal lesion is unknown, the patient usually is referred to a neurologist or neurosurgeon for further diagnosis and treatment. If the focal lesion has been diagnosed already and does not require specific treatment, the psychiatrist may treat the emotional or behavioral symptoms which brought the patient for psychiatric evaluation in the first place, with the knowledge that the brain lesion may both cause the symptoms and limit the patient's ability to cooperate with and benefit from therapy.

Patients in the third group, in whom dementia is uncertain, create more problems. Here the psychiatrist should turn to ancillary diagnostic tests (specifically psychologic testing, EEG, and computerized cranial tomography [CT-scan]) for assistance. Each may provide evidence to support a diagnosis of either focal or diffuse brain disease.

Psychologic testing often serves the psychiatrist well, but it should be recognized that when "the clinical assessment suggests doubtful impairment, psychologic testing usually produced equally doubtful results,"[17] Since the findings on psychologic testing that suggest organicity also occur in the pseudodementias, testing is most helpful in this group of patients when it is negative, i.e., when it provides no evidence that specifically suggests an organic defect. Stated differently, performance on psychologic testing can prove that a person is not demented; it can seldom if ever prove the presence of dementia when the clinical picture is uncertain.

The EEG is useful in these patients if it reveals either focal or diffuse dysfunction. It is not of much use if normal, for dementia may be advanced and the EEG remain normal.[31] The same is true for the CT-scan. If the CT-scan reveals a significant focal defect or moderate to severe diffuse atrophy, the physician can be secure in the diagnosis of organic disease. A normal CT-scan does not rule out dementia, however, since these are known to occur, especially in the reversible dementias.[3] On the other hand, the psychiatrist should not ascribe much importance to "mild" or "minimal" atrophy (as demonstrated by computed cranial tomography) in the face of clinical evidence in conflict with the diagnosis of dementia.[29] The significance of these lesser degrees of atrophy is unknown at present.

If the psychiatrist reached the fourth conclusion, i.e., that on the basis of history, mental status examination, and neurologic examination the patient has dementia most likely due to a diffuse disease process, an extensive diagnostic evaluation is called for, aimed at establishing a disease diagnosis on which a therapeutic program can be built.[25]

PROCEEDING TO A DISEASE DIAGNOSIS

Once dementia is established, a disease diagnosis must be achieved. In the past this has often been neglected, in the mistaken belief that no diseases that can be reversed or improved were likely to be uncovered. Recent studies demonstrate that this course of benign neglect is unwise.

Three series of patients with presumptive diagnosis of dementia have now been studied thoroughly neurologically for the identification of the specific underlying disorders.[4,9,15] These studies indicate that thorough medical evaluation results in diagnosis of potentially reversible disorders in approximately 15 percent. Reversible disorders include drug toxicity, normal pressure hydrocephalus, benign intracranial masses, mania, hypothyroidism, hyperthyroidism, pernicious anemia, folate deficiency, epilepsy, hepatic failure, and depression. In an additional 20 to 25 percent, disorders are uncovered in which specific therapeutic interventions are important, even though restitution to pre-existing cerebral integrity may be impossible. These measures include control of hypertension in multi-infarct dementia, palliative treatment for malignant brain tumors, withdrawal from alcohol in demented alcoholics, surgical treatment for normal pressure hydrocephalus to prevent progression even when brain damage cannot be reversed, antibiotics for neurosyphilis, and genetic counseling for families of patients with Huntington disease. In summary, thorough diagnostic evaluation uncovers disorders calling for treatment (other than symptomatic therapy) in 35 to 40 percent of patients who appear demented. Seltzer and Sherwin[21] reported that it is possible to achieve a disease diagnosis in virtually all patients who have been assigned a nonspecific neuropsychiatric diagnosis such as "organic brain syndrome."

The general physical examination is of special importance in the search for treatable causes of dementia. Do fever or stiffness of the neck suggest an infectious process? Is the blood pressure elevated pointing to multi-infarct dementia? Is the pulse irregular, suggesting multiple cerebral emboli? Does the appearance of the skin suggest anemia, polycythemia, jaundice, endocrine disorders, malnutrition, or lupus erythematosus? Does the breath smell of uremia or alcohol? Is there cardiomegaly, venous engorgement, peripheral or pulmonary edema to implicate cardiac failure in the genesis of the dementia? Pulmonary function is equally important—dyspnea, cyanosis, impaired respiratory movements, rales, and ronchi. Is the liver nodular or enlarged? Is there splenic or renal enlargement?

Many clues may emerge to point toward a specific diagnosis, but what if they do not? How does the physician then proceed? Obviously one cannot test for all possibilities, but what tests should be used routinely? Table 5-3 lists suggested diagnostic procedures for most patients with dementia for whom there are no clues to suggest specific diseases other than Alzheimer disease or senile dementia of the Alzheimer type. In the three series mentioned above, these tests alone, used routinely (in addition to clinical evaluation), would have uncovered all the treatable causes of dementia.

Many other diagnostic procedures may be appropriate in selected patients. The EEG and psychologic testing are two that are especially useful in certain instances, as is the examination of the cerebrospinal fluid. However, routine use of the procedures listed uncovers virtually all treatable disorders, and to add others to the protocol at this time would be unlikely to increase the yield significantly.

TABLE 5-3. Suggested laboratory studies for patients with dementia

Blood tests
   Complete blood count
   Serologic test for syphilis
   SMA-12, SMAC, or other standard metabolic screening tests
   Serum thyroxine by column (CT₄) or serum free thyroxine (FT₄)
   Serum B₁₂ and folate levels
Computerized cranial tomography
Urinalysis
Chest x-ray

Even the most meticulous study, however, fails in over half the cases of dementia to identify a specific disease, so that the patient is left without a disease diagnosis that can be confirmed. Excellent neuropathologic studies have demonstrated Alzheimer disease (or senile dementia of the Alzheimer type) to be the main cause of these diffuse atrophies,[22,23] and we believe it justified to make this diagnosis on clinical grounds in the middle-aged or elderly patient with: (1) chronic, progressive cognitive impairment by history; (2) evidence of diffuse dysfunction on mental status examination, with or without an abnormal neurologic examination; (3) evidence of moderate to severe diffuse atrophy by CT-scan; and (4) absence of clinical or laboratory features that permit the diagnosis of another specific causative disorder. An occasional error in diagnosis will doubtless occur, but the advantages of diagnosing Alzheimer disease clinically, especially in terms of treatment planning and family counseling, far outweigh the disadvantages.

TREATMENT

Specific therapy for the treatable disorders is detailed elsewhere.[25,27] We will discuss below only the therapeutic measures likely to be beneficial for all demented patients, whatever the underlying cause of their dementia.

The three basic aims in the symptomatic treatment of the demented patient are: (1) restitution of lost functions that are susceptible to restitution; (2) reduction of the patient's needs to use those functions that have been lost; (3) making the best use possible of residual functions.

Restitution of Lost Functions

This is accomplished mainly by correcting medical and physical problems. Demented patients are often thin and weak because their medical disorders, dietary needs, and exercise requirements have been neglected. Other treatment measures cannot be expected to help unless the patient is in the best possible physical condition. Prompt and thorough treatment of concurrent medical problems is even more important in demented patients than in others, for the diseased brain is especially vulnerable to the effects of fever, toxins, cardiac failure, pulmonary insufficiency, and renal dysfunction. The diseased brain is also vulnerable to the effects of deficient and distorted sensory perceptions; thus poor vision and deafness are special stresses for the already compromised brain. Eyeglasses and hearing aids may help significantly, and patients should be encouraged to use them. Demented patients often fail to eat unless the food is placed before them, and suffer as a result. Demented patients living alone will insist that they have eaten even though a check of the refrigerator reveals that no food has been consumed. An adequate dietary intake must be assured if other measures are to be effective. Exercise and physical therapy are important to keep the patients mobile as long as possible. The physical, psychiatric, and social problems of the patient confined to a wheelchair or bed are infinitely greater than those faced by the ambulatory patient.

Reduction of the Patient's Needs for Lost Functions

This is achieved largely through environmental manipulation, arranging the patient's situation and life so that he or she must confront inadequacies as little as possible. Thus patients must be protected from coming up against situations that are beyond their capabilities. Although stress may enhance performance in the healthy individual, stress is often severely disruptive to demented persons. Change is one variety of stress that may prove especially disruptive. Thus demented patients usually do best in quiet and familiar surroundings, with adequate but familiar distractions. Old friends and surroundings are therapeutic; new faces and new situations rather than being diverting are unusually upsetting. The darkness and quiet of nights may be particularly stressful, and a soft night light often provides help in orientation. If the patient must be moved to a hospital or nursing home, some cherished objects from home should be taken along to provide a sense of continuity and security.

Utilization of Residual Functions

To help the demented patient utilize the remaining brain functions fully, the physician may: (1) prescribe medications for relief of distressing symptoms; (2) provide directive and supportive psychotherapy; and (3) organize and integrate the various support systems providing care for the patient.

MEDICATIONS

Medications may be useful in the demented patient to: (1) reduce anxiety; (2) improve mood; (3) reduce paranoid and other psychotic symptoms; (4) control harmful behavior such as hyperactivity and assaultiveness; and (5) improve sleep. Treatment aims here not to restore lost functions but to create the best conditions possible for the utilization of remaining functions.

The use of any psychotropic agents in dementia requires caution. Sedatives usually are tolerated poorly; thus barbiturates and other hypnotic agents should be avoided. Because the diseased central nervous system is often exquisitely sensitive to psychotropic medications, small doses of these agents should be used initially. In general, response to psychotropic agents also is less predictable in the dementias than in functional disorders.

Chlordiazepoxide (Librium), 5 mg twice daily, or diazepam (Valium), 2 mg twice daily may be used initially for the control of anxiety. Dosage may be increased slowly to achieve better symptomatic relief.

For depression, the tricyclic antidepressants are used. There are no definite guidelines for the choice of specific tricyclics, but in general, amitriptyline and doxepin are reported to cause fewer cardiovascular side effects. In depressed patients with dementia, starting doses should probably be 10 mg three or four times daily, with gradual increases depending on clinical response and the development of side effects. Since many demented patients are also depressed, and since depressive pseudodementia may be difficult to distinguish from true dementia, a trial of therapy with the tricyclics should be considered in a sizable proportion of the demented patients encountered.

The antipsychotic agents are generally used for alleviation of paranoid and other psychotic symptoms and for control of potentially harmful behaviors. Chlorpromazine (Thorazine) or thioridazine (Mellaril) 25 mg two to four times daily, haloperidol (Haldol) 0.5 mg two or three times daily, or acetophenazine (Tindal) 20 mg two or three times daily may be tried initially. Chlorpromazine and thioridazine may have unwanted sedative and hypotensive effects, and while these are usually absent with haloperidol, this agent often produces extrapyramidal side effects. The piperazine phenothiazine derivative acetophenazine is reported to produce few extrapyramidal side effects and yet not too much sedation or hypotension in the organically impaired patient.[20] For the acutely disturbed patient 25 mg chlorpromazine by intramuscular injection is suggested, with subsequent treatment depending on initial response.

In patients with insomnia, promethazine hydrochloride (25 to 50 mg) at bedtime is often helpful. The sedating qualities of chlorpromazine and thioridazine can also often be used to promote restful sleep when given at bedtime.

Persons with dementia are vulnerable to delirium from any centrally active medication. Thus when a demented patient worsens "despite" taking psychotropic medications, the possibility should always be entertained that the worsening is caused by delirium resulting from the medication received.

PSYCHOTHERAPY

Although patients with dementia are obviously not candidates for insight oriented therapies, they can often benefit from supportive and directive techniques. Supportive therapy is used to help patients make the most effective use possible of the coping techniques and defense mechanisms at their disposal. Directive techniques are used to try to steer patients away from situations that are too demanding and toward situations where they still have the capacity to function. Thus the therapist encourages demented patients to continue their interests and simple social activities, to exercise, and to be productive in ways in which they can be appreciated by others as long as possible. At the same time the psychiatrist attempts to protect them from disruptive stresses and allows them to ventilate feelings of anger, fear, rejection, and hurt, in an atmosphere where such feelings are accepted and do not lead to rejection.

In the treatment of the demented patient, the needs of the family must also be considered. Three specific needs can usually be recognized: (1) assistance in recognizing and accepting the nature and severity of the disability; (2) assistance in planning and executing the specific treatment program that is best for the patient; (3) assistance in accepting the limits of what they and the physician can accomplish through any treatment program devised. Most families need help in all three of these areas. The psychiatrist also may play an important part in convincing guilt ridden family members to accept institutionalization of a demented member rather than turning the home into a hospital to no benefit to the patient.

ORGANIZATION AND INTEGRATION

Many people play roles in the care of the demented patient—family, physicians, nurses, social worker, physical therapist, friends, clergyman, recreational therapist, occupational therapist—and the role of each may be important. It is usually the physician's responsibility to organize and integrate the activities of these individuals, a difficult and often discouraging task, for the benefits of treatment often are not apparent in these disorders that steadily encroach on brain substance.

None of these measures aims directly to improve function of the diseased neurons. Although a number of medications from time to time have been reported to improve brain function per se, none has yet been reported to improve brain function consistently in the demented patient. At this time, Hydergine (a combination of three ergot preparations) probably has the most promise, coupled with considerable tolerance and safety in the demented patient. A trial of several weeks with 0.5 or 1.0 mg sublingually three times daily is probably warranted, especially in patients whose disease is not too far advanced who can cooperate in taking the medication.

Even with the best of treatment, the prognosis in dementia is poor.

Katzman[11] recently emphasized the "malignant" nature of Alzheimer disease, the most frequent of the dementing disorders. Life expectancy in this disorder is estimated to be reduced by 50 to 67 percent, based on the age at onset of symptoms. Kaszniak and associates[8] have presented further evidence that emphasizes the high mortality of patients with presenile and senile dementia. They also suggested that the degree of functional brain impairment may be the most important influence on mortality in these patients.

PSEUDODEMENTIA

Pseudodementia is the syndrome in which patients with functional psychiatric disorders present symptoms and changes on mental status examination that closely resemble those of true dementia. In the past, pseudodementia usually has been recognized in retrospect, after a patient has recovered unexpectedly instead of following a predicted downhill course. There is considerable evidence that this mimicry of dementia by functional psychiatric illness is not an unusual phenomenon, and consequently dementia is almost certainly overdiagnosed (especially in the aged). Patients in whom pseudodementia goes unrecognized stand, on the one hand, liable to superfluous, expensive, and possibly even dangerous diagnostic procedures and, on the other hand, in danger of therapeutic neglect through failure to diagnose and treat the underlying functional disorder.

Clinical Features

Pseudodementia can usually be differentiated from true dementia on the basis of history and mental status examination. The most consistently useful differentiating points are listed in Table 5-4.

HISTORY

When cognitive dysfunction has been relatively abrupt in its onset and is of short duration, pseudodementia should be suspected. As Kiloh noted in his classic paper,[13] an abrupt onset virtually rules out a diagnosis of dementia, which is usually insidious in onset and of long duration before medical attention is sought. On the other hand, many patients with pseudodementia present a time course not unlike that of dementia.[28] Patients with pseudodementia usually complain repeatedly of their memory loss (which is often one among many complaints), describe the loss in considerable detail, and report loss of both recent and remote memory. The typical patient with significant dementia, on the other hand, appears little aware and little worried about memory loss, and if the loss is recognized, it is described as most severe for recent events.

TABLE 5-4. Clinical features differentiating pseudodementia from dementia (Modified from Wells[28])

Pseudodementia	*Dementia*
1. Symptoms of short duration suggest pseudodementia	1. Symptoms of long duration suggest dementia
2. Patients usually complain much of cognitive loss	2. Patients usually complain little of cognitive loss
3. Patients' complaints of cognitive dysfunction usually detailed	3. Patients' complaints of cognitive dysfunction usually imprecise
4. Patients usually communicate strong sense of distress	4. Patients often appear unconcerned
5. Memory loss for recent and remote events usually equally severe	5. Memory loss for recent events more severe than for remote
6. Memory gaps for specific periods or events common	6. Memory gaps for specific periods unusual*
7. Attention and concentration often well preserved	7. Attention and concentration usually faulty
8. "Don't know" answers typical	8. "Near miss" answers frequent
9. Patients emphasize disability	9. Patients conceal disability
10. Patients make little effort to perform even simple tasks	10. Patients struggle to perform tasks
11. Patients highlight failures	11. Patients delight in accomplishments, however trivial
12. Patients do not try to keep up	12. Patients rely on notes, calendars, etc. to keep up
13. Marked variability in performing tasks of similar difficulty	13. Consistently poor performance on tasks of similar difficulty
14. Affective change often pervasive	14. Affect labile and shallow
15. Loss of social skills often early and prominent	15. Patients often retain social skills
16. On tests of orientation, patients often give "don't know" answers	16. On tests of orientation, patients mistake unusual for usual
17. Behavior often incongruent with severity of cognitive dysfunction	17. Behavior usually compatible with severity of cognitive dysfunction
18. Nocturnal accentuation of dysfunction uncommon	18. Nocturnal accentuation of dysfunction common
19. History of previous psychiatric dysfunction common	19. History of previous psychiatric dysfunction unusual

*Except when due to delirium, trauma, and seizures.

PSYCHIATRIC EXAMINATION

The suspicion of pseudodementia usually is raised on examination by the incongruence between the patient's complaints and the patient's performance (and by marked variability in different aspects of performance). The pseudodemented patient may, for example, complain insistently of poor memory and poor concentration, yet give a meticulously detailed history without faltering and without prompting. When asked for specific details, however, the pseudodemented patient often is quick with "I don't know" and "I can't remember" responses, giving the impression that little effort is expended in the search for the correct answer. Such responses are used to emphasize and confirm the patient's perceived incapacities. On mental status examination there also is often a marked and inexplicable (from an organic standpoint) variability in performance, with perhaps excellent performance on a difficult task, then total failure on a much simpler similar set of questions. In those patients who do not cooperate for a thorough mental status evaluation, marked inconsistency is often noted between their inability to respond to examination and their behavior otherwise, which may be clearly goal oriented and effective in attaining its objectives. Affective changes are often severe and pervasive in pseudodementia.

The demented patient, on the other hand, often denies or minimizes limitations in memory and concentration, even when these are grossly apparent to the examiner. In dementia, a variety of stratagems usually is employed to conceal the dysfunction; there is usually consistency in the defective performance; and behavior is in keeping with the severity of the manifested cognitive dysfunction. Affect is often shallow and labile.

In brief, there are usually striking differences on psychiatric examination between the demented and the pseudodemented patient, and the differential diagnosis rests predominantly upon the recognition of these differences.

Other Procedures

The neurologic examination is normal in pseudodementia, but it is often normal as well in dementia. The CT-scan is usually normal in pseudodementia but may also be normal on occasion in dementia. On the other hand, the CT-scan may be reported to reveal mild abnormalities when no dementia is present.[29]

We have found psychologic testing to be the most helpful of the ancillary diagnostic procedures. In pseudodementia, psychologic testing is usually characterized by marked variability in performance from one test to another, a variability which cannot easily be explained on the basis of either a focal cerebral lesion or diffuse cerebral atrophy. Correct interpretation of the test results requires considerable sophistication of the interpreting psychologist.

Psychiatric Diagnosis

We have emphasized thus far the clinical features that suggest to the examiner the syndrome of pseudodementia. The diagnosis can be accepted as a working hypothesis, however, only when a functional disorder giving rise to the syndrome has been identified.

Kiloh,[13] Post,[17] and Roth[19] all emphasized the importance of depressive illness, particularly in the elderly, in the production of the syndrome of pseudodementia. There is little question indeed that severe depressive disorders can produce a clinical state that almost exactly mimics dementia. Pseudodementia is not, however, limited to the affective disorders.[28] It may be a manifestation of chronic characterologic disorders (especially those in which severe longstanding dependency and a chronic depressive life style are intertwined), hysterical disorders, post-traumatic states, and schizophrenia. Almost certainly further study will identify other functional disorders which also give rise to pseudodementia.

Identification of the underlying psychiatric disorder is central in importance, for it is this diagnosis which leads to appropriate treatment. It is probably wise, in fact, to consider a diagnosis of pseudodementia as proven beyond doubt only when treatment has brought about disappearance of the pseudodementia (or when the pseudodementia is stationary in those cases in which treatment of the underlying chronic functional disorder is ineffective). In most cases, treatment results in a melting away of the manifestations even though the chronic characterologic symptoms may be resistant to change.

REFERENCES

1. American Psychiatric Association: Diagnostic and Statistical Manual of Mental Disorders, ed. 2. American Psychiatric Association, Washington, D.C., 1968.
2. Chapman, L.F., and Wolff, H.G.: The cerebral hemispheres and the highest integrative functions of man. Arch. Neurol. 1:357, 1959.
3. Fox, J.H., Topel, J.L., and Huckman, M.S.: Use of computerized tomography in senile dementia. J. Neurol. Neurosurg. Psychiatry 38:948, 1975.
4. Freemon, F.R.: Evaluation of patients with progressive intellectual deterioration. Arch. Neurol. 33:658, 1976.
5. Haase, G.R.: Diseases presenting as dementia, in Wells, C.E. (ed.): Dementia, ed. 2. F.A. Davis Company, Philadelphia, 1977.
6. Hachinski, V.C., Iliff, L.D., Zilhka, E., et al.: Cerebral blood flow in dementia. Arch. Neurol. 32:632, 1975.
7. Kahn, R.L., Zarit, S.H., Hilbert, N.M., et al: Memory complaint and im-

pairment in the aged. The effect of depression and altered brain function. Arch. Gen. Psychiatry 32:1589, 1975.

8. Kaszniak, A.W.; Fox, J.; Gandell, D.L., et al: Predictors of mortality in presenile and senile dementia. Ann. Neurol. 3:246, 1978.
9. Katzman, R.: Personal communication, 1975.
10. Katzman, R., and Karasu, T.B.: Differential diagnosis in dementia, *in* Fields, W.S. (ed.): Neurological and Sensory Disorders in the Elderly. Stratton Intercontinental Medical Book Corp., New York, 1975.
11. Katzman, R.: The prevalence and malignancy of Alzheimer disease: A major killer. Arch. Neurol. 33:217, 1976.
12. Kiev, A., Chapman, L.F., Guthrie, T.C., et al.: The highest integrative functions and diffuse cerebral atrophy. Neurology 12:385, 1962.
13. Kiloh, L.G.: Pseudo-dementia. Acta Psychiatr. Scand. 37:336, 1961.
14. Liston, E.H., Jr.: Occult presenile dementia. J. Nerv. Ment. Dis. 164:263, 1977.
15. Marsden, C.D., and Harrison, M.J.G.: Outcome of investigation of patients with presenile dementia. Br. Med. J. 2:249, 1972.
16. Paulson, G.W.: The neurological examination in dementia, *in* Wells, C.E. (ed.): Dementia, ed. 2. F.A. Davis Company, Philadelphia, 1977.
17. Post, F.: Dementia, depression, and pseudodementia, *in* Benton, D.F., and Blumer, D. (eds.): Psychiatric Aspects of Neurological Disease. Grune and Stratton, New York, 1975.
18. Roth, M., Tomlinson, B.E., and Blessed, G.: Correlation between scores for dementia and counts of "senile plaques" in cerebral grey matter of elderly subjects. Nature (Lond.) 209:109, 1966.
19. Roth, M.: Mental disorders of the aged: diagnosis and treatment. Med. World News Oct. 27, 1975, p. 35.
20. Salzman, C., Van Der Kolk, B., and Shader, R.I.: Psychopharmacology and the geriatric patient, *in* Shader, R.I. (ed.): Manual of Psychiatric Therapeutics. Little, Brown and Company, Boston, 1975.
21. Seltzer, B., and Sherwin, I.: "Organic brain syndrome": an empirical study and critical review. Am. J. Psychiatry 135:13, 1978.
22. Tomlinson, B.E., Blessed, G., and Roth, M.: Observations on the brains of demented old people. J. Neurol. Sci., 11:205, 1970.
23. Tomlinson, B.E.: The pathology of dementia, *in* Wells, C.E. (ed.): Dementia, ed. 2. F.A. Davis Company, Philadelphia, 1977.
24. Wells, C.E.: Dementia: definition and description, *in* Wells, C.E. (ed.): Dementia, ed. 2. F.A. Davis Company, Philadelphia, 1977.
25. Wells, C.E.: Diagnostic evaluation and treatment in dementia, *in* Wells, C.E. (ed.): Dementia, ed. 2. F.A. Davis Company, Philadelphia, 1977.
26. Wells, C.E.: Role of stroke in dementia. Stroke 9:1, 1978.
27. Wells, C.E.: Geriatric organic psychoses. Psychiatric Ann. 8:57, (Sept.), 1978.
28. Wells, C.E.: Pseudodementia. Am. J. Psychiatry 136:895, 1979.
29. Wells, C.E., and Duncan, G.W.: Danger of overreliance on computerized cranial tomography. Am. J. Psychiatry 134:811, 1977.
30. Willanger, R., Thygesen, P., Nielsen, R., et al.: Intellectual impairment and cerebral atrophy. A psychological, neurological and radiological investigation. Dan. Med. Bull. 15:65, 1968.
31. Wilson, W.P., Musella, L., and Short, M.J.: The electroencephalogram in dementia, *in* Wells, C.E. (ed.): Dementia, ed. 2. F.A. Davis Company, Philadelphia, 1977.

CHAPTER 6

HEADACHE AND FACIAL PAIN

Pain is probably the most common of all somatic symptoms, and pain of the craniofacial structures makes up a large portion of all pain problems. The term headache is used when pain involves the scalp or forehead, and the term facial pain is used when pain involves the facial area or the region in and around the nose and oropharynx. Virtually every person has experienced headache at one time or another, and migraine headaches in particular have been said to affect from 23 to 29 percent of the adult female and from 15 to 20 percent of the adult male population at some time.[21] Headache is, furthermore, the most common complaint in patients with primary psychiatric illness who are seen by neurologists for evaluation.[7] Entire books devoted to the complaint attest to its medical significance,[6,9,20,22] while a cursory inspection of television commercials attests to its ubiquitous interest for the common man.

Correct identification of the various disorders causing headache and facial pain is a prerequisite for management. Probably in no other clinical situation is the meticulous gathering and assessing of historical data so much more important than the physical examination and laboratory investigation for achieving an accurate diagnosis. Yet, unraveling an accurate history is difficult, because pain is such a personal experience that its character cannot be conveyed easily in words. Indeed, several interviews may be required to understand the character of the discomfort. In the majority of patients with headache or facial pain, the physical examination is entirely unremarkable.

The brain itself and its pia-arachnoid covering are insensitive to the usual painful stimuli. Structures that may give rise to pain include the basal dura, dural arteries, venous sinuses, vessels at the base of the brain, the fifth, ninth, and seventh cranial nerves, the nasal sinuses, and all extracranial structures. Pain may be caused by traction, pressure, or irritation of these sensitive structures.

The occurrence of headache or facial pain requires of the attending psychiatrist a high level of neurologic and medical sophistication. First, the psychiatrist must learn to recognize the commonly occurring pain syndromes so that, on the one hand, they are not mistakenly diagnosed as psychologic phenomena and, on the other hand, their relationship to underlying emotional stress and conflict may be appreciated. Second, the psychiatrist must be familiar with the appropriate medical treatment for the common pain syndromes, in order to manage the medical treatment directly (when concurrent treatment by internists or neurologists may be impractical or undesirable) and to appreciate the side effects of the medications used and their interactions with psychotropic agents. Lastly, the psychiatrist should learn to recognize those symptom complexes that merit or require extensive medical or neurologic investigation and those dealt with most appropriately by benign neglect. More than a mere smattering of knowledge is required.

Many medical illnesses give rise to cranial and facial pain as accompanying symptoms, but in this chapter we will focus largely on those disorders in which the major symptom is chronic or recurrent headache or facial pain. For our purposes we will use a modification of the classification proposed in 1962 by the Ad Hoc Committee on the Classification of Headache.[1]

RECURRING HEADACHE SYNDROMES

Vascular Headaches

CLASSIC MIGRAINE

In classic or typical migraine, the headache is preceded by neurologic symptoms which usually last 10 to 20 minutes. During the prodrome, vasoconstriction usually involves the blood vessels supplying one side of the brain and retina. The resulting symptoms involve the contralateral side and include scintillating scotomata in one or both eyes, scotomatous defects, hemianopsia, hemiparesis, unilateral sensory disturbances, aphasia, and dysarthria. Not all these symptoms are experienced by every patient; rather, each patient has a certain combination that tends to be unique and recurrent. The prodrome subsides only to be followed in several minutes by headache and nausea.

During the headache phase, dilation of branches of the external carotid artery occurs, usually confined to the hemicranium. The arterial walls are stretched, and the pulse amplitude is greatly increased. The headache is characteristically a unilateral throb, most intense in the temporal region. It increases in severity, peaks in about one hour, and lasts from four to five hours to several days. The pain is usually of high intensity. Anorexia, nausea, vomiting, photophobia, and phonophobia frequently accompany the pain and are often severe.

In the late stages of the headache, the pain often spreads to other regions of the head and changes in quality from a throb to a steady ache. During this late phase, edema develops in the walls of the dilated blood vessels and surrounding tissue with localized scalp tenderness. Tissue changes explain the change in character from a pulsatile throb to a steady ache accompanied by localized tenderness.

The biochemical events accompanying the typical migraine episode have attracted much interest in recent years, centering recently on the role of biogenic amines. The importance of biogenic amines in psychiatric disorders increases the psychiatrist's interest in the biochemical phenomena of the migraine attack. It is hypothesized that the prodromal phase is sparked by release of serotonin from platelet aggregations, resulting in cerebral vasoconstriction. The succeeding phase of vasodilation is less well understood. It may result in part from release of prostaglandin in response to a sudden elevation in serotonin, and it may be augmented by lower levels of serotonin resulting from its breakdown. Changes in vascular walls and perivascular tissues are known to be important factors in the localized swelling and lowered pain thresholds, but the exact mechanisms remain unclear. This topic has been reviewed recently.[8,16]

Classic migraine is usually a severe, prostrating, recurrent illness, much less frequent in occurrence than common migraine (described below). Classic migraine comprises probably no more than 10 to 15 percent of all vascular headaches. Sufferers of classic migraine commonly have a family history positive for similar headaches, although the exact mode of inheritance remains unclear. The headaches typically begin early in adult life and diminish in frequency during middle age, perhaps due to changes in hormonal functions. Evidence to support this explanation comes from the increase in frequency and severity of vascular headaches in women who take oral contraceptives and supplemental estrogen.

Although patients with classic migraine have often been described as compulsive, perfectionistic, overly conscientious, driving, and ambitious, these headaches occur in patients of all personality types and with various psychiatric illnesses.

COMMON MIGRAINE

The prodrome of common migraine is not associated with neurologic disturbances. Instead, common migraine may be preceded for hours or days by psychologic disturbances (irritability, depression, lassitude), gastrointestinal symptoms, or changes in fluid balance, but often there is no prodrome. The pain may be similar in location and character to that described for classic migraine, or it may be bilateral. Rarely it may be described as steady in nature rather than throbbing or aching. The headache often lasts longer than the classic type, and it is not always accompanied by nausea, vomiting, or photophobia. The common migraine headache is usually less predictable (in character, severity, and duration) for the individual patient than the headache of classic migraine. Probably 80 percent of all vascular headaches are of the common migraine variety.

CLUSTER MIGRAINE

Cluster migraine, also known by other names such as paroxysmal nocturnal cephalgia, migrainous neuralgia, histamine cephalgia, and Horton's headache, is predominately a male malady. It usually appears in middle age and tends to occur quotidianally for weeks to months, to be followed by a completely asymptomatic period lasting months to years before another cluster of headaches appears. There is no prodrome, and the patient characteristically is awakened abruptly by the headaches in the early morning hours. The pain reaches its peak within minutes, lasts for one to two hours, and ceases abruptly. The pain is constant and severe, being comparable in its intensity only to that produced by subarachnoid hemorrhage. It is unilateral and involves the orbitotemporal area, often being described as centered behind the eye. The patients typically pace the floor and not infrequently pound their heads against the wall. There is no nausea, but often there is ipsilateral flushing of the face, injection of the conjunctiva, tearing, nasal congestion, and, occasionally, ptosis and miosis.

COMPLICATED MIGRAINE

A migraine episode may be complicated by more serious neurologic symptoms. The timing of these symptoms in relation to the headache varies considerably. Most often they occur during the prodrome and cease before the onset of the headache (classic migraine), but at times they continue throughout or after the headache period, appear at the height of the headaches, or even occur in the absence of the headache per se. Rarely the neurologic deficits become permanent.

The most common symptoms are paresthesias involving one side of the body, beginning in a limb and spreading from there in a period of minutes. The more dramatic symptoms include hemiplegias and hemianopias, usually contralateral to the headache. When disturbances of extraocular or pupillary motility occur, the disorder is known as ophthalmoplegic migraine. Rarely aphasia, ataxia, confusion, or coma are seen. Children sometimes experience abdominal pain and nausea as a manifestation of migraine (abdominal migraine).

BASILAR ARTERY MIGRAINE[2]

This infrequent form of migraine typically is seen in young women. The

100

prodromal symptoms include bilateral visual loss and a variety of brain stem symptoms such as vertigo, ataxia, dysarthria, and bilateral paresthesias. The prodrome lasts for 10 to 20 minutes and is followed by a severe throbbing occipital headache with nausea and vomiting. The prodromal symptoms suggest disturbance of neurologic function in the territory supplied by the vertebrobasilar and posterior cerebral arteries, while the location of the headache suggests involvement of the occipital and posterior auricular arteries. The headache often occurs in relation to menstruation.

BENIGN ORGASMIC CEPHALGIA

Paulson and Klawans[15] described a variety of headache precipitated by orgasm. Psychiatrists should know this syndrome so that on the one hand it will not be confused with the much rarer and more severe headache due to subarachnoid hemorrhage during intercourse and on the other it will not be attributed to psychologic conflicts. These headaches usually begin with or just following orgasm, are of high intensity and of throbbing character, may be located in virtually any cranial region, last usually from a few minutes to a few hours, and may be recurrent. Most are believed to be vascular in origin because of the nature of the pain and the frequent family history of migraine. As a rule no treatment is required. Lance[10] described muscle contraction headaches also occurring during intercourse, usually in the preorgasmic phase. Less frequently, headaches beginning during intercourse may be due to low spinal fluid pressure; these patients experience the typical effect of posture on the pain that occurs with the postspinal-tap headache.

Muscle Contraction Headache

The most common nonvascular headache is known as muscle contraction or tension headache. There is no prodrome, but the onset is usually gradual and the progression insidious. The pain is usually bilateral, extending widely over the cranium, but the most common locations are occipitonuchal and frontotemporal. Although often described as a steady pain, the patient may not use the word pain at all, but rather may describe sensations of pressure, tightness, fullness, or a band-like discomfort. The headaches last hours, days, weeks, or even months, may be present continuously through the waking hours, and may recur frequently. They characteristically increase in intensity throughout the day and reach their peak in the early evening.

This type of headache is more common in middle age and afterwards. Patients who experience these headaches often are aware of varying degrees of anxiety, anger, frustration, depression, or fatigue, and they tend to ascribe the headaches to these feelings. The discomfort is generally attributed to sustained contraction of the scalp musculature, but it is difficult to account for all the observed features by this mechanism; it is likely that vascular changes, tissue hypoxia, and localized toxins play roles in the genesis of the discomfort as well. Muscle contraction headaches often occur along with migraine headaches, further complicating treatment efforts.

Hypertensive Headaches

Recurrent headaches are occasionally attributable to systemic arterial hypertension.[14] Typically the pain begins nocturnally, is present on awaking in the morning, and is located over the occiput. The pain is described as a deep ache which worsens with bending and straining and fades during the first several hours after rising. Traub and Korczyn[19] reported headache to be a complaint in nearly half the patients attending a hypertension clinic, being especially frequent in those with a systolic pressure over 170 mm Hg or with a diastolic pressure over 110 mm Hg. Control of the hypertension prevents recurrence of this variety of headache.

Nasal Sinus Obstruction

Congestion of the nasal sinuses by allergic or infectious sinusitis and anatomic obstruction to drainage can produce headache. Often the pain is located near the involved sinus, and there may be tenderness over the area. Involvement of the frontal sinus produces pain in the forehead, the maxillary sinus over the cheek, the ethmoid at the inner canthus of the eye, and the sphenoid sinus behind the eye. These headaches also may be aggravated by bending, stooping, straining, and other postural changes.

On examination the physician may find nasal stuffiness or drainage, fever, tenderness over the sinus, and darkness of the sinus to transillumination. Radiologic evidence of an obstructed sinus can help in making the diagnosis. Treatment is aimed at prompting drainage and attacking the underlying cause.

Functional Headaches

It must be acknowledged that a large number of recurrent headaches encountered in any diverse patient population fail to fit into any of the categories described above. Such headaches probably present a greater nosologic problem for psychiatrists than for other medical specialists, because psychiatrists usually try to define the psychologic mechanisms involved. In trying to classify these headaches, the psychiatrist is likely to confront a breakdown in nosology. Should they be considered conversion phenomena? Should they be regarded as delusional? Are they manifestations of an overweening hypochondriasis? For these headaches, there is no adequate conceptualization of the mechanism producing the discomfort, and the physician's unease in dealing with these symptoms often is increased thereby. In light of our present ignorance, it is perhaps best to classify them for the time being as "functional," i.e., headaches for which no pathophysicochemical basis has yet been uncovered, and best not to obsess as to whether they are hysterical or delusional or otherwise.

The functional nature of these headaches can usually be established by two observations: (1) failure of the headaches described to conform to any of the well established varieties described above or below and (2) descriptive features of the headaches themselves. Functional headaches are commonly described in such a fashion that their functional nature is easily recognized by the attuned ear, i.e., either they are described in terms so vague that they cannot be conceptualized, or in terms so dramatic that they defy belief, or in terms so bizarre that they are obviously psychotic. The lack of fit between these descriptions and those of the well established types of headaches whose pathophysiology is reasonably understood is obvious.

A confounding factor, of course, is that headaches due to physical dysfunction also occur in patients whose cognitive functions, personality characteristics, or psychosis result in descriptions that are vague, histrionic or bizarre. Caution is always indicated in diagnosing headaches as functional in such persons, especially when the headaches are a new complaint or when somatization is an unusual feature for the particular individual.

Headaches with Depression

The depressed patient often seeks medical help because of headaches. The depression may or may not be obvious, and close attention to the history and psychiatric examination is required for accurate diagnosis. The headache may take many forms; it may resemble common migraine, muscle contraction headache, or the headache due to an intracranial mass, or, more often, it may present with the characteristics of functional headaches described above. It knows no age limits. The essential diagnostic point is that the significance of the patient's depression and not the features of the headache itself be appreciated. Headaches per se rarely cause severe, pervasive depression. Causation much more often proceeds in the opposite direction, i.e., depression resulting in headache or depression being masked by headaches. Headaches due to depression respond to successful treatment or to spontaneous remission of the depressive episode.

NONRECURRING HEADACHES

A small but significant percentage of headaches is not chronic and recurrent over a period of years; these headaches generally have an identified beginning, a definite course, and an ending that is the result of appropriate treatment or of natural evolution. A brief description of some of the more important varieties of nonrecurring headaches is provided below.

Temporal Arteritis

Headache due to temporal arteritis assumes more importance than its incidence might warrant because of its imminent treatability and its disastrous outcome should it go unrecognized and untreated. Temporal arteritis is insidious in onset and usually occurs after the age of 50. The headache is unilateral, severe, throbbing, and of greatest intensity in the temporal region. The pain may be precipitated or exacerbated by chewing. The headache is accompanied or preceded by malaise, anorexia, weight loss, myalgias, and fever. The affected scalp arteries are nodular, thickened, and tender to palpation.

The mechanism is a giant cell arteritis of the external carotid artery and its branches.[3] The diagnosis is made on the basis of the typical clinical picture, an elevated erythrocyte sedimentation rate, and characteristic pathologic changes established by temporal artery biopsy. The illness is treated effectively with corticosteroids. Without treatment, there is danger of permanent loss of vision in one or both eyes. This condition is commonly misdiagnosed as depressive illness.

Post-traumatic Headaches

Often called the postconcussion syndrome, this type of headache frequently follows head injury of minor or major degree. The headache is commonly generalized but may present in many ways. It is usually only part of a complex syndrome whose components include anxiety, fatigue, disordered equilibrium, prolonged sleep, autonomic instability, difficulty with concentration, poor memory, irritability, and tearfulness (see Chap. 13). The whole syndrome may last a few days or linger for months. The mechanism involved is controversial; some believe that it results from structural damage, while others believe it to be a functional disorder resulting from anxiety and depression. Treatment consists largely of reassurance as to the benign nature of the disorder and its self-limiting course, but it must be conceded that this treatment is far from universally successful. When symptoms persist in patients without signs of significant neurologic dysfunction, a functional explanation for the headaches should be suspected.

Headaches Due to Intracranial Lesions

Headaches are common in subdural hematoma and brain tumor, but they are not so specific in character that they are diagnostic by themselves. With intracranial masses, the discomfort tends to be deep seated, either unilateral or bilateral, generally aching in character, and usually progressive in intensity, eventually becoming associated with established neurologic deficits or papilledema. They may awaken the patient at night and are often exaggerated by movements which increase intracranial pressure, e.g., stooping, bending, coughing, or sneezing.

Headaches due to intracranial aneurysms and arteriovenous malformations usually occur only after their rupture, with leakage of blood into cerebral subarachnoid spaces, although rupture intracerebrally can produce headache through traction and distension. Pain due to intracranial hemorrhage is acute, reaching its maximum within seconds or minutes, and is of high intensity. Only rarely can recurrent headaches be ascribed to such a lesion.

Headache also results from meningeal irritation. In acute irritation, such as that of bacterial meningitis or subarachnoid hemorrhage, the headache is acute in onset. With chronic meningeal irritation due to fungal, tuberculous, or neoplastic meningitis, the headache evolves over a few days or weeks. In both, the pain is deep seated, generalized, and associated with stiffness of the neck. The maneuvers mentioned above that increase intracranial pressure also exaggerate this type of headache.

TREATMENT OF HEADACHES

Many patients with headaches require no specific treatment. Often a simple explanation of the pathophysiology and assurance of the benign nature of the headaches are enough. In others, the headaches are so infrequent that treatment of the episode with analgesics and possibly bed rest suffices. If the patient can identify specific personal habits or environmental factors that precipitate headaches, the patient has a ready route to alleviate the headache. The patient should not, however, be encouraged too much in this pursuit, which tends frequently to become imaginative and far-ranging but unprofitable. With regret we conclude that only rarely can specific predictable precipitants (whether physical or emotional) be identified. The failure to identify precipitating events in no way argues against the importance of environmental and psychologic factors in the genesis of headaches in the headache prone individual; it only argues against a direct one-to-one relationship.

Vascular Headaches

Treatment of vascular headaches may be aimed either at relief of the individual episode or at its prophylaxis.[17] The mainstay of treatment for the individual episode is ergotamine tartrate, a vasoconstrictor which, if taken during the prodrome, often prevents the phase of scalp arterial dilation and headache. If no prodrome signals the impending headache, the medication, to be effective, must be taken at the first sign of a headache before the discomfort becomes too severe. Ergotamine tartrate can be administered sublingually, orally, rectally, by inhalation, or by injection. We have had greater success with the 2 mg sublingual form. The patient takes 2 mg initially and is allowed to repeat that dosage twice at 30 minute intervals. Regardless of the rate of administration, patients should be warned to avoid more than 6 mg in one day and more than 12 to 15 mg in one week. Failure to observe such restrictions can result in dangerous complications due to peripheral arterial constriction. Patients who are pregnant or have peripheral vascular disease should avoid ergot preparations altogether.

Regrettably, ergotamine tartrate is not always effective in aborting vascular headaches. When it is not, physicians generally rely on tranquilizers and analgesics to provide symptomatic relief. The major tranquilizers have proven useful, possibly because they also have antiemetic properties. Analgesics are often required, and sometimes narcotics must be employed. As in all chronic painful afflictions, the dangers of addiction must be constantly assessed.

For many patients, treatment of the individual episode is unsatisfactory, and prophylactic therapy is advisable. Saper[17] suggested a preventive approach: (1) when headaches occur so frequently that safety limits are exceeded for the medications used to treat the individual headaches; (2) when other medical conditions contraindicate use of medications used to abort headaches; and (3) when headaches occur with reliable regularity at specific times or under specific circumstances. The last situation can perhaps be dealt with easiest. When migraine attacks appear predictably, such as at certain times of the day or only on certain days, ergotamine tartrate may be taken prophylactically, within the daily and weekly limits for total dosage noted above.

In some patients, however, the frequency of migraine attacks is such that ergotism results if enough is taken to provide satisfactory relief or the ergot preparations are ineffective, not tolerated, or contraindicated, so that other preventive measures are sought. Daily administration of propranolol (Inderal) 20 to 40 mg four times daily, tricyclic antidepressants 75 to 200 mg nightly, clonidine hydrochloride 25 to 50 μg three times daily, or methysergide (Sansert) 2 mg three times daily have been reported to be effective in some patients. There are no guidelines as to which medication will prove effective in a specific patient. The incidence of fibrosis of retroperitoneal structures, pleura, and heart valves associated with long term administration of methysergide can be reduced by requiring a one month drug holiday every five months of usage. The very occurrence of such toxic reactions to ergotamine and methysergide speaks against their chronic administration in any but the most severe and refractory cases of vascular headaches.

Recently excitement has arisen concerning the use of relaxation and biofeedback techniques in the treatment of migraine; the predictability and duration of the benefit of these methods remain to be demonstrated. A frequent observation in the treatment of patients with vascular headaches is that new remedies prove effective *for a while* but then lose their effectiveness.

Treatment of cluster headaches is similar to that of classic migraine, although usually not as effective. If the headaches have a regular pattern, as they often do, ergotamine may be taken prior to the expected headaches (thus usually at bedtime). If a pattern is lacking or if ergotamine is ineffective, the medicines mentioned above may be tried on a regular daily basis. Recently maintenance therapy with lithium has also been reported to be effective in preventing cluster headaches.[4] However, the natural history of remissions and exacerbations of cluster headaches makes assessment of drugs difficult.

Nonvascular Headaches

In treating nonmigrainous headaches, the basic underlying pathophysiologic mechanism must be considered. Muscle contraction headaches may respond to measures that promote reduction of muscle activity, such as rest, massage, heat, and small doses of the minor tranquilizers. Headaches resulting from excessive muscle contraction are the variety which would be expected most reasonably to respond to relaxation and biofeedback techniques prompting muscle relaxation, and there is a growing list of publications to suggest the effectiveness of these methods in this disorder. Temporal arteritis requires corticosteroids. Hypertension induced headaches usually respond to an effective antihypertensive regimen. Post-traumatic headaches usually require no more than reassurance; at times they appear to respond to tranquilizers or antidepressants. The treatment of headache pain due to intracranial lesions and meningeal irritation is secondary in importance to treatment of the primary process.

Non-narcotic analgesics help reduce pain and suffering in virtually all the headaches discussed above in which the pathophysiology of the pain is understood. Non-narcotic analgesics by themselves, however, are virtually never sufficiently effective therapeutic agents in cases of severe recurrent headache. There is some question as to whether narcotic analgesics should ever be employed for chronic, recurrent headaches because of the danger of addiction. They might be used, however, for the patient with occasional severe, recurrent headaches if they can be shown to reduce morbidity significantly and if they are used only on a sporadic, infrequent basis.

Many patients with both vascular and nonvascular headaches of identified pathophysiology have been referred for psychiatric treatment (especially psychotherapy), usually after all other measures have failed. Martin[13] reported that 41 of 50 patients with tension headaches seen for psychiatric evaluation at the Mayo Clinic "revealed situations that were associated with grossly evident tension" and that most of the remaining nine handled conflict by denial. It is difficult to assess the results of psychiatric treatment in these patients, however, so many are the variables.

No mention has been made so far of treatment for functional headaches, i.e., those for which no specific pathophysiology can be identified. It is certainly safe to say that none of the measures described above aimed at the underlying pain mechanisms are likely to be effective in functional headaches except for a temporary placebo effect. There is likewise no proof that analgesics (narcotics or otherwise) are effective against these headaches, again aside from their placebo effect. The only effective treatment for functional headache is treatment directed toward the underlying psychiatric disorder. The effectiveness of psychiatric intervention thus depends on the treatability of the underlying disorder. When the headache is due to primary depressive illness, for example, treatment of the underlying depression is likely to result in cure both of the headaches and of the depression. When the headaches are associated with chronic schizophrenic disease or longstanding personality disturbance, psychiatric treatment would be anticipated to be less effective.

Much of the confusion about the effectiveness of all treatment modalities for headaches lies in the failure of most investigators to separate patients with functional headaches from those whose pathophysiologic mechanisms can be identified precisely.

FACIAL PAIN

Although less common than headache, recurrent pain limited to the face is not infrequent. The pain may be sensed entirely in the face or may be experienced in deeper structures such as the nose, mouth, and throat.

108

Recurrent facial pain is usually severe and may be either brief or prolonged. It may be limited to the distribution of a single cranial nerve; such pains are usually ascribed to neuralgias of the specific nerves. Other pains, similar in nature but not localized to the distribution of any specific nerves, will be discussed below as atypical facial pain.

Neuralgias

TRIGEMINAL NEURALGIA

Trigeminal neuralgia (also known as tic douloureux) is the most common of the neuralgias; it afflicts primarily middle-aged and elderly persons. The pain is sharp, lancinating, intense, unilateral, and paroxysmal. Each episode of pain lasts only seconds, but the episodes may occur from 1 to 100 times each day, sometimes being so close together that the pain seems constant. Between the attacks, there is no pain, and the neurologic examination is normal. Frequently, the pain is initiated by talking, chewing, or other movements, or by sensory stimulation of a certain area of the face or mouth by touch, food, or even a breeze. These sensitive areas are called trigger points. The second and third division of the trigeminal nerve may be involved either alone or in combination; the first division (supplying forehead and eye) is often involved but seldom involved alone. The pain can be so intractable and disabling that serious depression and even suicide ensue, yet the pain may remit spontaneously for months, years, or even permanently.

Medical therapy usually involves the administration of anticonvulsants—phenytoin (Dilantin) or carbamazepine (Tegretol). Analgesics are usually ineffective, and because of the severity and chronicity of the pain, addiction is a serious danger if narcotics are prescribed. In patients refractory to medical therapy, various surgical precedures have proved helpful, including alcohol or phenol injection of the affected nerve, electrocoagulation of nerve roots or ganglion, and manipulation or section of nerve roots next to the pons.

GLOSSOPHARYNGEAL NEURALGIA

This pain is similar in character to that of trigeminal neuralgia but is located in the area supplied by the glossopharyngeal and vagal nerves, i.e., the throat in the area of the tonsillar fossa, posterior part of the tongue, and rarely, in the ear. Triggering maneuvers include swallowing, chewing, talking, protruding the tongue, yawning, and laughing.

SPHENOPALATINE GANGLION NEURALGIA (SLUDER'S NEURALGIA)

This syndrome consists of pain in the roof of the nose, in and about the eye, in the upper jaws and teeth, and along the zygoma to the ear and mastoid area. The pain may be constant or paroxysmal. It is ascribed to inflammation of the sphenopalatine ganglion which is close to the ethmoid and sphenoid sinuses.

PARATRIGEMINAL NEURALGIA (RAEDER'S SYNDROME)

This syndrome is manifested by throbbing pain above one eye associated with nausea and vomiting. In addition there is partial or complete sympathetic dysfunction of the eye ipsilaterally, with miosis, ptosis, and decreased sweating in the brow area on the same side. Although most cases are idiopathic, some are accompanied by demonstrable lesions of the ipsilateral internal carotid artery, which carries the sympathetic nerves to the eye.

TREATMENT OF THE RECOGNIZED VARIETIES OF FACIAL PAIN

The treatment of all the facial neuralgias is similar to that described for trigeminal neuralgia. Anticonvulsant medicines such as phenytoin (Dilantin) and carbamazepine (Tegretol) are prescribed initially. If they are unsuccessful and disabling pain persists, often the specific nerve root involved may be subjected to surgical treatment (injection or sectioning). Even in the typical forms of facial pain, antidepressants may be useful even if serious depression is not apparent clinically. Whether this response is due to effective therapy for a masked depression or whether the tricyclic antidepressants have another pharmacologic effect in these neuralgias is unknown.

Temporomandibular Joint Syndrome (Costen's Syndrome)

A degenerative process of the temporomandibular joint can be the cause of intermittent or constant pain at the site of the joint in front of the ear, often with radiation of the pain to the temple and jaw. There may be a clicking sound or crepitation in the joint. In many instances the etiology is thought to be dental malocclusion. The pain of Costen's syndrome is typically less severe than the forms of neuralgia considered above.

Other, even rarer, causes of facial pain include: *occipital neuralgia,* which provokes pain in the occipital, suboccipital, and parietal regions of the scalp (within the distribution of the greater occipital nerve); *neuralgia of the geniculate ganglion* (VII cranial nerve), which causes pain in the external auditory canal and pinna of the ear and may be associated with vesicles of herpes zoster in the painful area and with facial palsy (Ramsay Hunt syndrome); *herpes zoster of the gasserian ganglion* (V cranial nerve), which is associated with severe pain and herpetic eruption in the distribution of the trigeminal nerve, particularly its first division.

Atypical Facial Pain

Much, some might say most, severe recurrent facial pain does not fit into the well defined categories described above. Nevertheless, enough homogeneity exists among these pain problems, which do not conform to classic patterns, so that they have come to be grouped together as atypical facial pain.[5,11,12,18] It is the identity of the overall clinical presentation rather than the identity of the pain pattern per se which leads to this classification.

The patient with atypical facial pain who is seen by the psychiatrist virtually always has had the pain for many months or years. Most are middle-aged women. The pain often began after some minor and apparently uneventful dental or surgical procedure involving the face, teeth, tongue, or throat, and from such a trivial beginning the discomfort has grown in all dimensions so that now it virtually engulfs the patient. The pain has usually spread to involve large segments of the lower-half facial and cranial structures, mainly unilaterally but at times crossing the midline. It has increased in duration and severity, so that whether steady or paroxysmal, the pain persists throughout most of the patient's waking hours; it is usually described as the most severe pain conceivable. Although usually characterized as throbbing, aching, or lancinating, not infrequently it is described in theatrical or bizarre terms. Many factors may trigger or accentuate the pain.

The patient almost invariably sees the psychiatrist as a last resort and usually with great reluctance. He or she likely has consulted internist, dentist, neurosurgeon, otolaryngologist, and neurologist (often in multiples), has tried many treatment modalities to no avail, and is convinced of the organic genesis of the pain. Medical, neurologic, and dental examinations have proved unfruitful. Whatever traces of pathology that have been uncovered are insufficient to account for pain of such magnitude, and remedies aimed toward these trivial disorders have more often seemed to lead to worsening than to relief. Usually the patient has become withdrawn and overtly depressed, unable to focus attention for any significant period on anything other than the pain, and perceiving this as the logical consequence of pain so intense and so persistent.

Authorities are unanimous in ascribing virtually all examples of atypical facial pain to psychiatric causes, primary depressive illness being the most generally accepted etiology. Unfortunately, identifying the basis as psychiatric does not lead uniformly to successful treatment.

111

Although good results have been reported in some patients treated with antidepressants, many patients angrily reject psychiatric intervention. Even the best psychiatric treatment is ineffective in many of those patients who willingly cooperate, especially in those whose pain persisted for long periods before treatment was begun. Early diagnosis and early psychiatric intervention are essential for an acceptable outcome.

THE PSYCHIATRIST'S ROLE IN EVALUATING HEADACHE

Many patients with headache or facial pain are referred for psychiatric evaluation and treatment; many patients under psychiatric care have headache chronically or develop them in the course of treatment. These complaints often present perplexing problems for the psychiatrist. Not every patient can be sent to a neurologist for assurance that the headaches are not due to intracranial disease. Yet psychiatrists must gauge how thoroughly an intracranial lesion or medical etiology has been excluded in patients referred for psychiatric treatment of their headaches. They must also decide what measures, if any, are required to rule out these possibilities in psychiatric patients with intercurrent headaches.

No protocol will be applicable in every instance. Nevertheless, several features should alert the psychiatrist to the possibility that a serious medical cause exists. One should always be wary when an adult who has not previously been subject to headaches begins to suffer significantly incapacitating head pains. One should be equally wary when the headache prone adult begins to experience severe headaches of a new and distinctly different character. The complaint of one patient with severe recurrent migraine that a particular headache was not like any she had ever had before led to the diagnosis of a pheochromocytoma. Another signal for caution is the presence of headache that does not appear to fit with the rest of the clinical picture. Thus a complaint of severe headache in a patient who appears to have an acute schizophrenic psychosis should alert the physician to a possible diagnosis of encephalitis. A headache that is initially mild and intermittent but gradually over days or weeks becomes constant and severe causes special concern. Recurrent, episodic headaches seldom result from intracranial disease processes.

Analysis of the character of the pain is often helpful. A deep aching pain is usual with intracranial pathology; throbbing or lancinating pains are atypical for intracranial disease processes. Headache due to an intracranial mass is often most severe on awakening (or may wake the patient from sleep) and abates in the course of the day. Headache which is significantly modified by changes in posture, movement, coughing, sneezing, or straining is often secondary to intracranial disease.

Any serious headache warrants thorough medical and neurologic examination. When, as is so often the case, these uncover no cause for the headache, how far should the search be pursued? Every patient with headache cannot have skull X-rays, electroencephalogram, and CT-scan, but if not in every patient, in which are they indicated? In trying to provide acceptable guidelines, one should note that when the history does not suggest a focal neurologic lesion and when a meticulously performed neurologic examination is entirely within normal limits, it is unlikely that any of these diagnostic procedures will provide an explanation for the headache. When these clinical features are lacking, further neurologic diagnostic procedures are indicated only if the course or character of the headache strongly suggests the likelihood of an intracranial lesion. However, when the history suggests a focal lesion or when the neurologic examination is abnormal, further diagnostic procedures should always be pursued. The psychiatrist must follow the clinical cues rather than approach the problem with any set formula.

Negative ancillary diagnostic studies provide little reassurance to either patient or physician except when the nature of the headache did not suggest a serious medical disorder or intracranial lesion in the first place (in which case ancillary diagnostic procedures were probably not indicated anyway). When the character of the patient's headaches suggests that they are not benign, however, negative studies are interpreted by neurologists to indicate only that the offending cause has not been identified, not that a serious cause will not eventually be uncovered.

Lastly, as in all instances of somatic distress, we would caution psychiatrists not to accept a psychiatric etiology for a patient's headache or facial pain without other specific evidence of psychiatric dysfunction. The psychiatrist should never accept the proposition that if no organic cause for the discomfort can be identified, it must therefore be psychiatric in origin. When thorough and sensitive psychiatric evaluation reveals no evidence of significant psychiatric dysfunction in the patient with headache or facial pain, the psychiatrist should state so clearly and not accept the patient for treatment. There are patients with headache and facial pain whose discomfort we cannot explain satisfactorily on either a physical or psychiatric basis; they deserve further study and observation, not spurious categorization.

REFERENCES

1. Ad Hoc Committee on the Classification of Headache: Classification of Headache. JAMA 179:717, 1962.

2. Bickerstaff, E.R.: Basilar artery migraine. Lancet 1:15, 1961.
3. Cooke, W.T., Cloake, P.C.P., Govan, A.D.T., et al.: Temporal arteritis: A generalized vascular disease. Quart. J. Med. 15:47, 1946.
4. Ekbom, K.: Lithium in the treatment of chronic cluster headaches. Headache 17:39, 1977.
5. Engel, G.L.: Primary atypical facial neuralgia. An hysterical conversion symptom. Psychosom. Med. 13:375, 1951.
6. Freidman, A.P., and Merritt, H.H.: Headache: Diagnosis and Treatment. F.A. Davis Company, Philadelphia, 1959.
7. Kirk, C., and Saunders, M.: Primary psychiatric illness in a neurological out-patient department in north east England. Acta Psychiatr. Scand. 56:294, 1977.
8. Kudrow, L.: Current aspects of migraine headache. Psychosomatics 19:48, Jan. 1978.
9. Lance, J.W.: The Mechanism and Management of Headache, ed. 2. London, Butterworth, 1973.
10. Lance, J.W.: Headaches related to sexual activity. J. Neurol. Neurosurg. Psychiatry 39:1226, 1976.
11. Lascelles, R.G.: Atypical facial pain and depression. Brit. J. Psychiatry 112:651, 1966.
12. Lesse, S.: Atypical facial pain of psychogenic origin: A masked depressive syndrome, in Lesse, S. (ed.): Masked Depression. Jason Aronson, New York, 1974.
13. Martin, M.J.: Tension headache: A psychiatric study. Headache 6:47, 1966.
14. Moser, M., Wish, H., and Freidman, A.P.: Headache and hypertension. JAMA 180:301, 1962.
15. Paulson, G.W., and Klawans, H.L., Jr.: Benign orgasmic cephalgia. Headache 13:181, 1974.
16. Saper, J.R.: Migraine. I. Classification and pathogenesis. JAMA 239:2380, 1978.
17. Saper, J.R.: Migraine. II. Treatment. JAMA 239:2480, 1978.
18. Smith, D.P., Pilling, L.F., Pearson, J.S., et al.: A psychiatric study of atypical facial pain. Can. Med. Assn. J. 100:286, 1969.
19. Traub, Y.M., and Korczyn, A.D.: Headache in patients with hypertension. Headache 17:245, 1978.
20. Vinken, P.J., and Bruyn, G.W. (eds.): Headaches and Cranial Neuralgias. North-Holland Publishing Company, Amsterdam, 1968 (Handbook of Clinical Neurology, vol. 5).
21. Waters, W.E., and O'Connor, P.J.: Prevalence of migraine. J. Neurol. Neurosurg. Psychiatry 38:613, 1975.
22. Wolff, H.G.: Headache and Other Head Pain. Revised by D.J. Dalessio (ed. 3). Oxford University Press, New York, 1972.

CHAPTER 7

EPILEPSY

Epilepsy is the most common chronic neurologic disease. Because of its frequency, it once was and now should be the most important area for cooperative patient study and treatment between neurologists and psychiatrists. The advent and proliferation of anticonvulsant medications have resulted, however, in epilepsy's falling almost entirely into the purview of neurologic specialists, and the behavioral problems of epileptic patients have gone largely unattended. Blumer[3] wrote: "Neurologists, by nature of their interest and training, tend to pay little attention to the psychologic symptoms in epileptics. Psychiatrists on the other hand tend to overlook the epileptic nature of certain mental changes, or—once the diagnosis is known—often shun epileptics as cases from an alien field."

Yet there is little question that the incidence of behavioral and emotional disorders is high in epilepsy. A significant number of epileptic patients are hospitalized, briefly or chronically, on psychiatric inpatient units, and every neurologist is aware of the behavioral and psychologic problems of epileptic patients, even though these may not be a focus of treatment. Pond[21] recently reviewed the epidemiologic studies dealing with the incidence of psychiatric disturbances in epilepsy. From the data that he assembled, it appears that at least 30 percent of all epileptics (children and adult) have significant psychiatric difficulties. Rodin[22] placed the incidence even higher, at nearer 50 percent. Furthermore, the frequency and type of psychiatric disturbance varies from one type of epilepsy to another. Psychosis is more frequent, for example, in epilepsy of temporal lobe origin, and although there is not a consensus, many believe that the impairment caused by behavioral disturbances is greater in temporal lobe epilepsy as well.

The psychiatrist should learn about epilepsy for at least three reasons: (1) to recognize and diagnose epilepsy and to separate it from functional disorders simulating epilepsy; (2) to deal therapeutically with the psychiatric problems complicating epilepsy; and (3) because the study of epilepsy throws light on the neural bases of behavior.

DEFINITION

Defining the term epilepsy to the satisfaction of all is impossible. Most would agree that the terms epilepsy and seizure disorder are similar if not synonymous, and in practice the terms are used interchangeably. Epilepsy tends to connote chronicity, the tendency to have recurring or repeated seizures, and the presence of some ongoing, underlying brain dysfunction. Thus, a patient with a single seizure related to some specific medical event would *not* be said to have epilepsy.

The phenomenon of seizures or epilepsy is an old one. Some date it as far back as the Code of Hammurabi, and most credit Hippocrates, in his work *On The Sacred Disease* in 400 B.C., with identifying epilepsy as a disease of the brain. Initially, largely unscientific, superstitious, and supernatural theories were invoked to explain the clinical phenomena. A modern scientific view was introduced by Thomas Willis and later by Hughlings Jackson, who defined epilepsy as a group of disorders with paroxymsmal and excessive neuronal discharge that caused a sudden disturbance in neurologic function. This 1870 definition by Jackson has not seen subsequent major alteration or improvement.

CLASSIFICATION

Many approaches to classification of the different types of seizures have been made. Terms such as grand mal, petit mal, Jacksonian seizures, temporal lobe seizures, and psychomotor seizures have become familiar medical terms but have led, in some instances, to confusion because of different meanings given to these terms by different people. Recently, an attempt to unify and clarify classification has been made with the establishment of the International Classification of Epileptic Seizures.[10] However, even this classification has not been accepted and endorsed uniformly by those who work in the field.

In this chapter we utilize a modification of the international scheme which we have found clinically useful (Table 7-1). Many of the types of seizures are not important to the psychiatrist in daily practice and will be mentioned only briefly. Those seizures arising from temporal lobe foci and, less often, from inferior frontal foci are of considerable importance to the psychiatrist and will be discussed in some detail.

GENERALIZED SEIZURES

When a seizure is called generalized, the implication is that there is a

TABLE 7-1. Classification of seizures

I. Generalized seizures
   A. Tonic and/or clonic seizures (grand mal)
   B. Absence seizures (petit mal)
   C. Bilateral myoclonus
   D. Infantile spasms
   E. Atonic seizures

II. Partial seizures
   A. Simple partial
      1. Motor seizures (includes jacksonian)
      2. Sensory seizures
      3. Affective
   B. Complex partial seizures (psychomotor seizures)

III. Unclassified seizures

lack of evidence to suggest a focal origin. There is no aura or prodrome to indicate abnormal function of a particular part of the brain, and there is no focal electroencephalographic abnormality. The electroencephalogram (EEG) records a seizure pattern developing in a generalized distribution, appearing in leads from both hemispheres simultaneously. It is not certain if the abnormality appears in both hemispheres because it is projected from a deeper midline source or if both hemispheres become involved simultaneously because of some humoral or systemic abnormality; the former theory is favored currently.

Tonic/Clonic Seizures (Grand Mal)

The typical grand mal seizure is the type most familiar to physicians. It can serve as a model in the description of its component parts, which will then be applicable to the description of other types of seizures. A grand mal seizure may consist of the following components (although not all are invariably present): prodrome, aura, ictus, and postictal state. For several hours, or in some instances several days, prior to a seizure the patient may have a vague feeling of discomfort or anxiety which is usually characteristic enough that it can be predicted that a seizure will occur soon. This state, called the prodrome, is not clearly understood but is not thought to represent effects of increased abnormal electrical discharges in the brain. At the beginning of the paroxysmal discharge that constitutes the seizure itself, before consciousness is lost, the patient may become aware of an unusual bodily sensation often described as a numbness rising up from the epigastrium, a sensation of faintness, or turning of the head and eyes. This brief period, called the aura, is thought to represent the remembered part of the seizure, and the aura is properly considered a part of the seizure itself. Its characteristics are probably related to the anatomic origin of the seizure, and its occurrence suggests the possibility that the seizure has a focal origin. Only about half the patients with grand mal seizures have such an aura.

The ictus itself begins with tonic extension of all four extremities and often with arching of the back and neck. This correlates with the paroxysm of spikes in the EEG. The tonic phase soon gives rise to clonic activity, which may be thought of as tonic extension alternating with relaxation of the muscles; this phase is correlated with the appearance on the EEG of alternating spikes and slow waves. Fecal and urinary incontinence often occur. The ictus usually lasts 1 or 2 minutes but can be prolonged. During this phase, the patient is unconscious.

Following the period of clonic activity, the postictal phase, which varies from patient to patient, begins. Some patients regain consciousness almost at once with only minimal symptoms of fatigue or headache; others experience varying degrees of unconsciousness or stupor, lasting from minutes to hours, often accompanied by headache, confusion, and fatigue. After the seizure, the patient may remember the aura, if one occurred, but does not remember the period of convulsive movements. Memory may also be lost for portions of the postictal period. If the patient was alone or asleep at the time of the seizure, he or she may be totally unaware of its occurrence or may only find evidence of the seizure such as clothing soiled with urine or feces or a bitten, sore tongue.

Absence Seizure (Petit Mal)

Absence seizures usually begin between the ages of 5 and 7 years and usually cease by the time of puberty. The absence seizure is characterized by a brief interruption of consciousness during which time the patient abruptly ceases whatever activity he or she may have been doing and loses awareness of what is going on in the environment. During the spell, the patient may blink the eyelids or smack the lips but does not fall to the ground or have convulsive movements of the arms and legs. The spells usually last only 2 to 10 seconds.

The EEG is distinctive and characteristic, consisting of regular, repetitive spike-and-wave complexes at a frequency of three per second. This patterned discharge is present in most patients during the seizure and usually is elicited easily during the interictal period with activation by hyperventilation or photic stimulation. The paroxysmal spike-and-wave complexes appear simultaneously and symmetrically on both sides of the brain and are thought to be caused by a focus discharging in the diencephalon, thus the alternative name centrencephalic epilepsy.

In some instances, however, the absence seizure disorder may extend into or rarely even have its onset in late adult life, causing considerable diagnostic difficulty.[8,13,26,27] The diagnostic difficulty arises because in this age group the patients may not experience the typical absence episodes described above, but the seizure disorder may make its clinical appearance under the guise of an acute psychotic episode, delirium, or a prolonged confusional or stuporous state. The EEG may reveal continuous diffuse three per second spike-and-wave activity, but protracted generalized 1.5 to 2 Hz spike-and-wave activity also may be observed.[8] Wells[27] pointed to four clinical features that suggest an epileptic etiology: (1) the abrupt onset of psychosis in a person regarded heretofore as psychologically healthy; (2) delirium unexplained by more common etiologic factors; (3) a history of similar episodes with abrupt spontaneous exacerbations and remissions; and (4) a history of fainting or falling spells. Making the correct diagnosis is especially important because effective treatment is available, and additional episodes may be prevented by appropriate long term anticonvulsant therapy.

The seizures termed bilateral myoclonus, infantile spasms, and atonic seizures are less common and usually occur in infancy and childhood. These will not be discussed here, and the reader is referred to standard neurologic textbooks if additional information is needed.

PARTIAL SEIZURES

The term partial seizures implies seizures which have an onset of focal origin, i.e., seizures which begin with only a part of the brain involved with epileptiform activity. Oftentimes the epileptic activity remains confined to the focus of origin or its nearby surroundings, and the patient remains conscious. At other times, the epileptic activity spreads from the focus to involve the entire brain, thus becoming indistinguishable clinically and electroencephalographically from generalized seizures. The interval between the onset of the focal paroxysm and the generalized spread varies considerably. In some instances, it is easy to diagnose focal seizures with generalized spread from the history, when observers can describe two distinct phases to the seizure—that is, first restricted symptoms suggesting a focal paroxysm and then a generalized tonic/clonic seizure. At other times the interval between focal onset and diffuse involvement may be so brief that it cannot be discerned even by an experienced observer; in these cases it is often the EEG which demonstrates the focal origin of the seizure. Generalized spread may follow either simple or complex partial seizures.

Simple Partial Seizures

When partial seizures consist of elemental neurologic symptoms, e.g., focal motor or focal sensory symptoms, the term simple partial seizures is used. The ictal manifestations of all partial seizures depend upon their site of origin. The most common form is a focal motor seizure which results from an epileptic focus in the contralateral frontal lobe. The seizure may consist of convulsive movements limited to a limb or part of a limb, or the movements may spread after beginning focally or "march" to involve the entire limb, the entire ipsilateral side of the body, and the contralateral side of the body as well. This particular sequence of spread has been termed a Jacksonian seizure. Usually by the time both sides of the body are involved, the patient has lost consciousness. On the other hand, the motor manifestations may be limited to a turning of the head and eyes to the side opposite the discharging focus; these are called adversive seizures. If a focal motor seizure remains confined to one group of muscles and lasts for a prolonged period of time (hours to days), the term epilepsia partialis continua is appropriate; this is the equivalent of focal status epilepticus.

Other simple partial seizures are less common. Epileptogenic foci in the anterior parietal lobe give rise to focal sensory seizures. The parts of the body involved are similar to those in focal motor epilepsy, but with focal sensory seizures the patients experience unusual sensations such as paresthesias, pins-and-needles, or numbness. When the site of origin is in the language area, the usual manifestation is speech arrest or muteness (see Chap. 2); however, in rare instances the patient may suddenly produce paraphasic or jargon speech (ictal aphasia). An epileptic focus in the visual cortex usually produces nonformed, elemental visual sensations such as lines, dots, or lights. More formed visual images have been described with foci in the posterior medial temporal lobe. Olfactory hallucinations, usually unpleasant and vaguely described odors such as burning rubber or dead fish, indicate a focus in the inferior medial aspect of the temporal lobe in the region of the uncus. Vertiginous sensations and auditory hallucinations are even rarer and probably result from foci within the temporal lobe.

Complex Partial Seizures

This group of partial seizures is termed complex because, although the origin is still focal, the clinical manifestations of the seizure discharge are more complex and elaborate, involving alterations of behavioral, mental, somatomotor, sensory, and autonomic functions. The terms complex partial seizures and psychomotor seizures are essentially synonymous, but it is not correct to equate these two terms with the term temporal lobe seizure. Although most complex partial seizures have their origin in the temporal lobe, some are known to originate in the frontal lobe, especially on its inferior surface.

Many patients with a temporal lobe focus present with a history of generalized convulsions alone, presumably because the latency between onset of focal discharge and its generalized spread is so short that a more elaborate seizure pattern is never recognized. Other patients have definite symptoms and signs of a complex partial seizure which are then followed by a generalized convulsive state. These generalized manifestations do not detract from calling them complex partial seizures.

Complex partial seizures typically have four components: sensory, psychic, autonomic, and somatomotor. The sensory components are usually vague but are described in such terms as giddiness, auditory distortions, visual aberrations (such as micropsia or macropsia), unusual tastes, or disagreeable odors.

The psychic symptoms are those that set this seizure type apart and make it of special interest to psychiatrists. These symptoms are complex and varied, and a complete description of them cannot be provided here. Among the many psychic symptoms described are feelings of impending disaster, altered states of awareness in seemingly alert patients (strangeness, depersonalization, abnormal clarity of perception), dreamy states and twilight states, forced thoughts, hallucinations (often complex), and sensations of déjà vu (familiarity in unfamiliar settings) and jamais vu (unfamiliarity in familiar settings), Taylor[24] and others have highlighted the resemblence between many of these psychic epileptic symptoms and those of schizophrenia.

The autonomic symptoms, not distinctive to this disorder, include palpitations, piloerection, nausea, increased salivation, dry mouth, hunger pangs, and even abdominal pain.

The somatomotor component is made up largely of automatisms, i.e., movements or acts without conscious volition. Automatisms usually take the form of movements about the facial-oral area such as blinking of the eyes, grimacing, lip smacking, chewing, spitting, or swallowing. Other stereotyped repetitive movements may occur such as gesturing, rubbing, patting, undressing, and wiping or wringing of the hands. The somatomotor phase is more difficult to recognize as an ictal phenomenon than is the tonic-clonic phase of the generalized convulsion, and problems not infrequently arise in differentiating this ictal event from a psychogenic phenomenon. The somatomotor phase usually lasts only seconds, rarely over 1 to 2 minutes. The movements tend to be repetitive, inappropriate, and fragmented. Only rarely do the movements make up elaborate or complicated acts, and there are few verified cases in which patients have carried out extended elaborate acts during an actual seizure. Violence and aggressive behavior are unusual as ictal events, and even more rare are directed, seemingly organized aggressive acts.

Typically, the patient experiences the sensory components initially, and this experience of the aura is often well remembered. The next phase is usually that of psychic abnormalities, and it varies widely from patient to patient. These symptoms are usually remembered, but less clearly than the initial sensory symptoms. Well formed visual or auditory hallucinations may occur, as well as visual and auditory,illusions or distortions. A patient may experience so-called dyscognitive states with sensations of unreality and detachment or, more characteristically, déjà vu or jamais vu sensations. Emotional or affective states, such as extreme happiness, pleasure, depression, fear, or (very rarely) rage may also be components of this phase of the seizure itself.

Following the stage of psychic symptoms, the patient may regain full consciousness, develop generalized convulsions, begin the somatomotor phase as described above, or enter a postictal period of unresponsiveness.

After a generalized convulsion, the postictal state may persist for minutes to hours. During this period, the patient is usually to varying degrees unrousable, disoriented, and confused, and amnesia of some extent is common for the period of postictal obtundation. In the absence of a generalized convulsion, the postictal phase of disturbed cerebral function usually is not long. Complex motor phenomena such as driving from one city to another, with complete amnesia for the act, have been described occasionally in the postictal state, but this is extremely rare. Prolonged "fugue states" during which the subject behaves in an orderly, normal fashion are almost always nonorganic in origin.

Relationship Between Complex Partial Seizures and Behavioral Abnormalities

Although there is no consensus as to its exact type or origin, most experienced clinicians agree that there are behavioral alterations in patients with complex seizures and that these changes are related both to the occurrence of the seizures themselves and to their site of origin. Psychologic abnormalities are not limited, of course, to patients with complex partial seizures, but in patients with generalized seizures and simple partial seizures, these are attributed largely to cognitive defects and to the psychosocial stresses to which epileptic patients are subject. Two primary types of change have been described in complex partial seizures: (1) interictal behavioral and personality changes,[1-3,21,25] and (2) interictal schizophrenia-like psychoses.[5,9,12,23]

INTERICTAL PERSONALITY CHANGES

Interictal behavioral and personality changes generally make their appearance several years after the onset of temporal lobe epilepsy. The patients are said to develop a deepening of all emotions. They take everything seriously, lose all sense of humor, and become unusually concerned about morals and frequently hyper-religious. They grow excessively concerned about details and often develop hypergraphia, keeping elaborate notes and diaries about the minutiae of everyday life. With this, they acquire a quality that has been called viscosity, i.e., a hanging on to others with words and details which often creates uneasiness and discomfort in those around them. Despite these changes, they are often described as good natured and warm individuals, sufficiently attractive that family and friends tolerate them for their good points despite the problems that these personality changes create otherwise.

Hyposexuality is common. This is more often an absence of interest in sexual activity than an inability to perform the sex act. Patients who develop temporal lobe epilepsy before puberty often fail to gain interest in sex when puberty occurs, and those who develop temporal lobe epilepsy after puberty often lose their former zest for sexual activity.

The behavior of these patients also is often marked by irritability and impulsivity. Outbursts of angry behavior develop in many of them, and at times their behavior may be verbally abusive and physically destructive. These outbursts tend to occur after periods during which the patient has pent-up anger and envy. Blumer[3] stated that these outbursts of violence (1) occur on provocation, although the provocation may be slight; (2) are directed toward the environment; (3) lack stereotypy; (4) are not associated with other seizure phenomena; (5) are remembered (although amnesia may be feigned); and (6) are often looked back on with remorse. These episodes of violence thus lack all the criteria for complex partial seizures. In this regard, Geschwind[11] wrote: ". . . many clinicians are likely to assume that amnesia for an episode of behavior disorder is evidence supporting temporal lobe epilepsy while the absence of amnesia for such an episode is against temporal epilepsy. Our experience would disagree strongly with this view. Temporal lobe epileptics typically remember their episodes of behavior disorder and claim amnesia only under special circumstances, such as the threat of prosecution."

Bear and Fedio[2] studied the personality characteristics of temporal lobe epileptics as described by the patients themselves and by observers. Temporal lobe epileptics scored themselves as humorless, dependent, and obsessional; observers rated them as circumstantial, philosophical, and angry. Those with right temporal lobe foci were scored as more "emotive;" those with left, as more "ideative." Bear[1] hypothesized that "the mechanism of interictal changes likely involve progressive modification of limbic structure secondary to a limbic lobe focus." Blumer[4] suggested "the syndrome of temporal hyperconnection in epilepsy" as a term for these personality changes.

Most of the personality changes described are believed to have little relationship to the effectiveness of seizure control. Most studies appear to have been carried out, however, in patients whose seizures were under relatively poor control. The "global hyposexuality" is, however,

123

closely correlated with poor seizure control, and adequate control of seizures, whether achieved by medical or surgical means, often leads to normalization of sexual interest and activity in these patients. It is said, on the other hand, that good control of complex partial seizures often leads to increased irritability and aggressiveness.[4]

Whether these interictal qualities are peculiar to seizure patients with temporal foci has not been established. It is rare for any single patient with temporal lobe epilepsy to manifest all the qualities described above, and in general neurologic practice many temporal lobe patients are encountered in whom these behavioral characteristics are not apparent even after thorough questioning. Geschwind[11] noted also that other personality constellations are seen in temporal lobe epilepsy as well. The relationship of the interictal behavioral qualities to the more severe schizophrenia-like illnesses remains to be elucidated.

SCHIZOPHRENIA-LIKE PSYCHOSES

The second major psychiatric abnormality reported in temporal lobe epileptics is schizophrenia or schizophrenia-like psychosis with an incidence several times that seen in the general population. These psychotic manifestations tend to begin typically 15 or more years after onset of temporal lobe epilepsy. Pincus and Tucker[20] pointed out that because of this long interval, there is in virtually all these patients a history of prolonged use of anticonvulsant medications; consequently the possible etiologic role of anticonvulsants in these psychoses has been debated.

Although these patients exhibit many typically schizophrenic phenomena, especially paranoid features, they differ in several important ways from most patients with schizophrenia. They develop psychotic changes later in life, lack a family history of psychosis, maintain good rapport with others and good affectual modulations, and do not in general suffer a schizophrenic form of deterioration. In addition, Glaser[12] wrote that the continued efforts to maintain contact with reality along with the lack of autism, archaic thinking, withdrawal, or peculiar symbolism set this disorder apart from the usual schizophrenic psychosis. Slater and associates[23] emphasized that in their follow-up studies many of these patients with the passage of time came to appear less schizophrenia-like and more organic-like.

Both Taylor[24] and Flor-Henry[9] emphasized that these schizophrenia-like psychoses do not just occur at random among temporal lobe epileptics; psychosis is more likely in females and in those with temporal lobe foci on the left. Flor-Henry[9] also emphasized the "epileptic" nature of the psychosis, and in his carefully controlled study, "the presence of psychomotor seizures and frequent temporal fits" was inversely correlated with the presence of psychosis. Thus Flor-Henry's patients were most psychotic when their complex partial seizures were best controlled.

(In another carefully controlled study, Kristensen and Sindrup[15] also found complex partial seizures to be significantly less frequent in their psychotic than in their nonpsychotic patients with temporal lobe epilepsy.) Glaser,[12] however, was unable to establish this inverse relationship between psychosis and seizure frequency and EEG abnormalities in his series of patients with interictal psychosis, although the inverse relationship was noted in a few of them. Kristenson and Sindrup[16] observed, on the other hand, that EEG epileptiform abnormalities were both more extensive and more severe in their psychotic than in their nonpsychotic group. They believed deep temporal lobe dysfunction to be a significant factor in the pathogenesis of psychosis in temporal lobe epilepsy.

DIFFERENTIAL DIAGNOSIS

In most patients, the diagnosis of epilepsy is easily made on the basis of clinical manifestations. This statement is not true, however, for many of the patients whom the psychiatrist is asked to see, because in many of these there will be a question about whether the spells are epileptic or functional in origin[8,17,26,27] (the latter have been called pseudoseizures by Liske and Forster[18]). The problem is compounded by the well known frequency with which hysterical spells are observed in patients with well established epilepsy.

The most marked diagnostic confusion is likely to arise in patients suspected of having complex partial seizures. Although grand mal, petit mal, and simple partial seizures are sometimes mimicked by hysterical spells, they are not often mimicked very successfully, so that diagnostic confusion is minimal. The situation is strikingly different, however, with the vast number of clinical manifestations described for complex partial seizures. Pincus and Tucker[20] suggested six questions to help distinguish complex partial seizures from transient aberrations due to hysteria or psychosis:

1. Does the patient describe subjective changes typical of complex partial seizures?
2. Has the patient been observed performing any of the characteristic automations?
3. Was the patient confused during the episode?
4. Was the patient's memory impaired for events during the episode?
5. Did the patient experience a postictal period of impaired thinking or depression?
6. Has the patient had other lapses during which he or she manifested nearly identical behavior?

The answer to these questions is usually yes in patients experiencing repeated complex partial seizures.

Several other points should be noted in any discussion of the differentiation of epilepsy from episodes of psychogenic origin. The physician should not let the bizarreness of clinical manifestations weigh too heavily on the side of a functional diagnosis, because epileptic seizures are often bizarre. The six questions listed above are a much better guide to diagnosis than the appearance of the episode per se. Nor should the physician let the influence of environmental events on the occurrence and the pattern of a spell speak too much against a diagnosis of epilepsy. Environmental events of affectual significance to the patient not infrequently precipitate an epileptic seizure or have some bearing on the clinical manifestations of the epileptic seizure itself. Liske and Forster[18] observed correctly, however, that "when both precipitant and seizure are unusual, the diagnosis of pseudoseizures is probable." We emphasize again that complex partial seizures are *very* rarely manifested by a period of amnesia during which the patient performs complicated and well organized acts successfully and without apparent difficulty.

The electroencephalogram is often helpful in differential diagnosis, particularly when the discharges typical of epilepsy are present. A negative EEG is not, however, so helpful. Kiloh, McComas, and Osselton[14] stated, for example, that single routine EEG records may be normal in 20 to 30 percent of patients with epilepsy. Although the yield of positive EEGs can be increased by a variety of techniques such as sleep recordings and sphenoidal electrodes, there nevertheless remain patients with epilepsy in whom an abnormal EEG is never obtained. This may be because the EEG is never recorded at a time when epileptic discharges are occurring, or perhaps because the recording electrodes cannot be placed where they can pick up the abnormal activity. In any event, normal interictal EEGs never preclude the diagnosis of epilepsy, although a normal EEG recorded at the time of a spell is strong evidence against organicity.

ETIOLOGY

In general, seizures are considered either to be due to some primary disorder of the brain, i.e., idiopathic epilepsy, or to be symptomatic of some other illness (Table 7-2). Symptomatic seizures may be further divided into those in which the brain is structurally changed by some identifiable disease process and those in which brain function (but not structure) is transiently disturbed by a metabolic derangement.

Taken in the larger sense, idiopathic epilepsy includes seizures occurring in any age group without apparent etiology. A more restricted use of the term idiopathic epilepsy refers to those seizure types which begin in childhood and teenage years and are probably inherited. These types include the generalized tonic-clonic and absence seizures. While most

TABLE 7-2. Etiology of seizures

I. Idiopathic (autosomal dominant inheritance?)

II. Symptomatic
    A. Structural
       Neoplasm, stroke, trauma, arteriovenous malformation, abscess, congenital
       defect, birth injury, degenerative disease.

    B. Metabolic
       Hypoglycemia, hyperglycemia, drug and alcohol withdrawal, acute anoxia,
       uremia, hypocalcemia, hypomagnesemia.

    C. Occult

authorities would agree that there must be *some* type of brain lesion, none has yet been identified. When generalized or partial seizures begin after the teenage years, they are considered symptomatic, and a thorough diagnostic evaluation depends on the type of seizure experienced, the age of onset, and general medical and neurologic examinations. If no etiology can be found, one should not be content to apply the term idiopathic and dismiss further thoughts as to etiology. On the contrary, the physician should consider the lesion *occult* and possibly identifiable at a later time.

The genetics of epilepsy is still unclear. None of the recognized modes of inheritance adequately explains the high incidence of clinical seizures in relatives of epileptics. Large scale EEG studies of the relatives of epileptics with absence seizures indicate that the EEG abnormality is inherited in an autosomal dominant mode, but the incidence of clinical seizures in these relatives is far less than would be expected if the seizure disorder were inherited in this manner.[19] This discrepency between the incidence of the EEG abnormality and its expression as a clinical seizure disorder is not understood.

TREATMENT

The treatment of epilepsy involves more than the use of anticonvulsant medications. If the seizures are found to be symptomatic of some other illnesses, primary therapy should be directed toward them, and treatment of the seizures themselves becomes secondary.

Anticonvulsant medications should be kept as simple as possible. The aim is to abolish the seizures using the fewest and the safest drugs possible. In general, one anticonvulsant is begun at a time, and the dosage is gradually increased until maximal therapeutic serum levels are reached before a second medication is added. The choice of medication depends in large measure on the seizure type. If satisfactory control is not reached or if a breakthrough occurs after good control has been achieved, the serum level should be checked before increasing the dosage or adding other drugs. If the serum level is low, simple encouragement to conform to the medication schedule or increasing the dosage of the medication usually suffices. An important point to remember is that the fewer medications prescribed and the simpler the schedule of their administration, the better is patient compliance. Tables 7-3 and 7-4 present information about the choice of anticonvulsants, usual dosages, and therapeutic serum levels.

The clinician often is faced with treating the patient who has both verified epileptic seizures and pseudoseizures. Whenever the number of spells increases in tandem with increasing doses of anticonvulsants, the possibility that the worsening is due to pseudoseizures should be considered. As Blumer[4] observed, increased anticonvulsants result in cerebral toxicity which leads to further regression and to increased pseudoseizures. In these cases, the aim is to treat the epilepsy with the smallest amounts of anticonvulsants possible and to treat the pseudoseizures with benign neglect.

Much of the treatment of epileptics is directive. Epileptics and their families should be encouraged to lead as normal lives as possible. Par-

TABLE 7-3. Indications for specific anticonvulsants

Tonic-clonic seizures
    Phenytoin (Dilantin)
    Phenobarbital
    Carbamazepine (Tegretol)

Absence seizures
    Ethosuximide (Zarontin)
    Clonazepam (Clonopin)
    Valproic Acid (Depakene)

Partial seizures, simple and complex
    Phenytoin
    Primidone
    Carbamazepine

TABLE 7-4. Anticonvulsant drugs, dosages and therapeutic serum levels

Drug	Dosage (mg/kg)	Serum level (µg/ml)
Phenytoin	4-7	10-20
Phenobarbital	1-5	20-40
Primidone	10-25	8-12
Tegretol	7-5	6-10
Ethosuximide	15-35	50-90
Valproic Acid	15-30	40-100

ents often need to be reminded that the child must be taught self-sufficiency in order to live a satisfactory adult life. Regular participation in physical activities should be encouraged, even though some precautions need to be taken, e.g., avoiding swimming alone. On the other hand, the physician has the obligation to warn the patient of the potential danger of driving automobiles, working around dangerous machinery, and going into dangerous places. All epileptic patients should be encouraged to follow regular schedules, eat adequately, get sufficient rest, and avoid alcohol and other drugs. Recent years have seen a growth of community resources for epileptics, such as vocational rehabilitation efforts and comprehensive epilepsy centers.

Psychiatric evaluation and treatment is requested with increasing frequency for epileptic patients. More effective anticonvulsants and better overall seizure control make it apparent that these patients have many behavioral and emotional problems that cannot be attributed to recurrent seizures alone. At this time, epileptic patients are seen by psychiatrists most frequently because of outbursts of angry aggressivity which make their management at home or in sheltered environments difficult. These angry and sometimes destructive outbursts may or may not be associated with psychosis. As noted above, in the case of complex partial seizures, it is possible that more effective seizure control actually leads to an increase in angry outbursts and psychosis.

Several neurologists and psychiatrists have recently addressed the treatment of these disorders.[4,5,7,12,21,22] The basic approach is a medical one. Blumer[4] called attention to the chemical structural similarity between carbamazepine (Tegretol) and the antipsychotic phenothiazines and the tricyclic antidepressants. He stressed that not only is carbamazepine an effective anticonvulsant, but it often results in striking improvement in behavior. Unfortunately, the administration of carbamazepine is not without its dangers, not only hematologically, but it is at times followed by profound worsening of behavior and psychotic manifestations.

Antipsychotic agents are the mainstay of treatment for both the angry aggressivity and the schizophrenia-like psychosis of epilepsy. Their efficiency has been amply demonstrated. Although some of these agents lower the threshold for seizures in experimental animals, this should not deter the psychiatrist from prescribing them when they are indicated. The danger of increasing seizure frequency is slight. There is no consensus as to which antipsychotic medication is most effective. Detre and Feldman[7] suggested use of fluphenazine (Prolixin) in a dose range between 6 and 20 mg daily. In none of their 16 patients did simultaneous administration of fluphenazine and anticonvulsant drugs cause an increase in the seizure frequency or severity. Blumer[4] reported the use of a variety of antipsychotic drugs—haloperidol (Haldol), thioridazine (Mellaril), trifluoperazine (Stelazine)—in these patients with improvement in behavioral symptoms and with no increase in seizures.

Although antipsychotics are the basic treatment modality in these patients and may be a prerequisite for treatment with other modalities, they are not sufficient when used alone. Psychotherapy is important for most of these patients. It may take the form of directive therapy, supportive therapy, or even at times insight oriented therapy. Blumer[4] detailed its effectiveness in one patient with temporal lobe seizures whose interictal personality changes had caused grave difficulties in interpersonal relationships. In addition, psychiatric hospitalization is often valuable, for crises in some and for long-term management and rehabilitation efforts in others.

Most epileptic patients will continue to be cared for primarily by neurologists, and so they should be. Nevertheless, the role of the psychiatrist in selected patients is an important one, and it may well prove to be an expanding one as better control of the seizures is achieved.

REFERENCES

1. Bear, D.: The significance of behavioral change in temporal lobe epilepsy. McLean Hosp. J. Special Issue, June 1977, p. 9.
2. Bear, D., and Fedio, F.: Quantitative analysis of interictal behavior in temporal lobe epilepsy. Arch. Neurol. 34:454, 1977.
3. Blumber, D.: Temporal lobe epilepsy and its psychiatric significance, *in* Benson, D.F., and Blumer, D. (eds.): Psychiatric Aspects of Neurologic Disease. Grune & Stratton, New York, 1975.
4. Blumer, D.: Treatment of patients with seizure disorder referred because of psychiatric complications. McLean Hosp. J. Special Issue, June 1977, p. 53.
5. Bruens, J.H.: Psychoses in epilepsy, *in* Vinken, P.J., and Bruyn, G.W. (eds.): Handbook of Clinical Neurology, vol. 15. North-Holland Publishing Company, Amsterdam, 1974.
6. Davison, K., and Bagley, C.R.: Schizophrenia-like psychoses associated with organic disorders of the central nervous system: a review of the literature. Brit. J. Psychiatry Special Publication No. 4:113, 1969.
7. Detre, T., and Feldman, R.G.: Behavior disorder associated with seizure states: Pharmacological and psychosocial management, *in* Glaser, G.H. (ed.): EEG and Behavior. Basic Books, Inc., New York, 1963.
8. Ellis, J.M., and Lee, S.I.: Acute prolonged confusion in later life as in an ictal state. Epilepsia 19:119, 1978.
9. Flor-Henry, P.: Psychosis and temporal lobe epilepsy. A controlled investigation. Epilepsia 10:363, 1969.
10. Gastaut, H.: Clinical and electroencephalographical classifications of epileptic seizures. Epilepsia 11:102, 1970.
11. Geschwind, N.: The clinical setting of aggression in temporal lobe epilepsy, *in* Fields, W.S., and Sweet, W.H. (eds.): Neural Bases of Violence and Aggression. Warren H. Green, Inc., St. Louis, 1975.
12. Glaser, G.H.: The problems of psychosis in psychomotor temporal lobe epileptics. Epilepsia 5:271, 1964.

13. Goldensohn, E.S., and Gold, A.P.: Prolonged behavioral disturbances as ictal phenomena. Neurology 10:1, 1960.
14. Kiloh, L.G., McComas, A.J., and Osselton, J.W.: Clinical Electroencephalography, ed. 3. Appleton-Century-Crofts, New York, 1972.
15. Kristensen, O., and Sindrup, E.H.: Psychomotor epilepsy and psychosis. I. Physical aspects. Acta Neurol. Scand. 57:361, 1978.
16. Kristensen, O., and Sindrup, E.H.: Psychomotor epilepsy and psychosis. II. Electroencephalographic findings (sphenoidal electrode recordings). Acta Neurol. Scand. 57:370, 1978.
17. La Wall, J.: Psychiatric presentations of seizure disorders. Am. J. Psychiatry 133:321, 1976.
18. Liske, E., and Forster, F.M.: Pseudoseizures: A problem in the diagnosis and management of epileptic patients. Neurology 14:41, 1964.
19. Metrakos, K., and Metrakos, J.D.: Genetics of convulsive disorders. II. Genetic and encephalographic studies in centrencephalic epilepsy. Neurology 11:474, 1961.
20. Pincus, J.H., and Tucker, G.J.: Behavioral Neurology, ed. 2. Oxford University Press, New York, 1978.
21. Pond, D.A.: Epilepsy and personality disorders, in Vinken, P.J., and Bruyn, G.W. (eds.): Handbook of Clinical Neurology, vol. 15. North-Holland Publishing Company, Amsterdam, 1974.
22. Rodin, E.A.: Psychosocial management of patients with seizure disorders. McLean Hosp. J. Special Issue, June 1977, p. 74.
23. Slater, E., Beard, A.W., and Glithero, E.: The schizophrenia-like psychoses of epilepsy. Brit. J. Psychiatry 10:95, 1963.
24. Taylor, D.C.: Epileptic experience, schizophrenia and the temporal lobe. McLean Hosp. J. Special Issue, June 1977, p. 22.
25. Waxman, S.G., and Geschwind, N.: The interictal behavior syndrome of temporal lobe epilepsy. Arch. Gen. Psychiatry 32:1580, 1975.
26. Weissberg, M.P.: A case of petit-mal status: A diagnostic dilemma. Am. J. Psychiatry 132:1200, 1975.
27. Wells, C.E.: Transient ictal psychosis. Arch. Gen. Psychiatry 31:1201, 1975.

CHAPTER 8

NEUROPSYCHIATRIC SEQUELAE OF CHRONIC ALCOHOL ABUSE

Psychiatrists are better acquainted than neurologists with many of the neuropsychiatric complications of chronic ethanol abuse, e.g., alcoholic hallucinosis and pathologic intoxication. We will not discuss these syndromes here, but we will consider only those complications that generally are considered more neurologic than psychiatric in nature but are nevertheless likely to be encountered by the practicing psychiatrist. We will not deal with those neurologic sequelae such as peripheral neuropathy or toxic amblyopia that are unlikely to pose problems for psychiatrists.

DISORDERS OF ALCOHOL WITHDRAWAL

Several distinct clinical syndromes have been noted to follow alcohol withdrawal. Usually at least several days, and often many weeks, of steady consumption of alcohol in large amounts has set the stage for the development of symptoms. The withdrawal is not necessarily abrupt and total but can be only a significant reduction in alcohol intake. Thus the patient may still have measurable ethanol in the blood when the symptoms begin. The withdrawal or abstinence syndrome consists of the following elements, either singly or in various combinations: tremulousness, hallucinosis, seizures (rum fits), and delirium tremens.

Tremulousness and Hallucinosis

Tremulousness usually occurs following an evening of abstinence and consists of a rapid (6 to 8/sec), coarse tremor which is prominent during willed movements. This tremor is often referred to as "nerves" and can be quieted temporarily by another drink or two. Usually accompanying the tremulousness are anxiety, anorexia, nausea, and vomiting. Also during this period, the patient may experience unusual sensitivity to

133

sounds and lights and ascribe to them unusual interpretations or ani-mation. Disturbing nightmares are frequent and become incorporated into the events of awake experiences. Auditory and visual hallucina-tions, often accusatory, may occur but are distinguishable from delirium tremens by their brief duration and the lack of other symptoms of delirium.

Alcohol Withdrawal Seizures[8]

Alcohol withdrawal seizures (rum fits) follow a predictable course. They appear without warning during a period of relative or absolute absti-nence, often after several hours of tremulousness or hallucinations. They may occur in spree drinkers or in more chronic alcoholics but always follow a protracted period of alcohol abuse. In Victor's series,[8] the two shortest periods of consecutive drinking that culminated in seizures were five and seven days.

Ninety percent of all withdrawal seizures occur between 7 and 48 hours after cessation of drinking, with the majority in the 12 to 24 hour period. The seizures are usually generalized tonic-clonic in type without focal features. Most patients experience a single seizure, but a short series of convulsions is not unusual. When multiple seizures occur, they usually take place within a period of six or so hours. Status epilepticus is rare.

Wikler and associates[11] demonstrated electroencephalographic ab-normalities, usually paroxysmal in nature, that were especially promi-nent during the 24 to 48 hours following alcohol withdrawal. Electroen-cephalograms that are obtained on these patients at other than the period of withdrawal are usually normal. During the two or three days following withdrawal, these alcoholic patients (both those with and without seizures) often demonstrate remarkable sensitivity to photic stimulation. Repetitive photic stimulation frequently provokes repeti-tive myoclonic jerks and abnormal electroencephalographic discharges, sometimes culminating in a clinical seizure.

Victor[8] emphasized particularly the role of alcohol consumption and its withdrawal in the genesis of alcoholic seizures. Patients with alco-holic seizures almost certainly would not have convulsions were it not for their alcohol abuse. They did not suffer seizures before they began to abuse alcohol; they do not come from families that have an increased incidence of epilepsy; and, as noted above, they usually have normal electroencephalograms except for the period immediately following the reduction in alcohol consumption (whereas the interictal EEG is ab-normal in a large percentage of patients with other varieties of epilepsy).

On the other hand, alcohol may also play a role in the occurrence of seizures in patients who have true epilepsy. Some patients who have idiopathic or symptomatic epilepsy become alcoholic or from time to time abuse alcohol, and alcoholics frequently suffer cranial trauma which results in post-traumatic epilepsy. Withdrawal from alcohol lowers the seizure thresholds and precipitates seizures in these patients as well, but these patients make up a small minority of the alcoholic patients who have convulsions, and they should not be diagnosed as having alcoholic seizures per se. The magnitude of the role that alcohol plays in seizures can be gauged from the study of Earnest and Yarnell.[4] Of a large number of adults admitted to a city hospital because of seizures, they found a history of alcohol abuse in 41 percent.

Alcohol withdrawal seizures usually require no specific therapy. When repeated seizures or status epilepticus occurs, the patient is treated with intravenous diazepam or barbiturates as in other types of seizure disorders. Theoretically, alcohol seizures might be preventable, were each patient protected with anticonvulsant medications for the first 48 to 72 hours after drinking is stopped or reduced, but there are no good studies available to show how effective this might be. Greenblatt and Shader[5] suggested that the benzodiazepines are the preferred agents for treating the symptoms of the alcohol withdrawal syndrome (for details, see Chap. 3), and because the benzodiazepines also possess anticonvulsant properties, their use probably provides some degree of protection against alcoholic seizures. In theory, phenothiazines might be contraindicated in the period immediately following alcohol withdrawal, because they might precipitate convulsions in patients whose seizure threshold has already been lowered as a result of the alcohol withdrawal. In fact, however, these agents are used routinely to treat the alcohol withdrawal syndromes in some institutions, without evidently increasing the incidence of alcohol withdrawal seizures. [This does not impugn the safety of the antipsychotic agents when they are prescribed to control behavioral symptoms in patients with epilepsy who are also being treated with maintenance anticonvulsants (see Chap. 7).] Patients who experience seizures only after alcohol withdrawal should not be treated with long term maintenance anticonvulsants. The dangers, both of poor compliance and of combining ethanol with anticonvulsants, in this group of patients outweigh its possible prophylactic value.

Delirium Tremens

Delirium tremens is one of the many varieties of delirium covered in detail in Chapter 3; here we will emphasize only a few of its aspects. Delirium tremens results from alcohol withdrawal, and it must be distinguished from the many other types of delirium that may occur in alcoholic subjects—those due to acute or chronic ethanol intoxication, thiamine deficiency, hepatic failure, hypoglycemia, head injury, acute sepsis, and dehydration. It is usually an agitated, excited delirium accompanied by frightening hallucinations, but it cannot be differentiated with certainty on the grounds of its clinical manifestations alone from deliria due to other causes occurring in alcoholics.[12]

Delirium tremens is set apart diagnostically from other deliria only by its predictable relationship to alcohol withdrawal. The first 24 to 48 hours off alcohol are marked by the nonspecific symptoms (tremulousness) of alcohol withdrawal and, in some, by alcoholic seizures. Delirium tremens usually makes its appearance two to four days (or even longer) after the patient stops drinking, its symptoms and signs sometimes seeming to grow out of the nonspecific symptoms or to emerge out of a period of postictal confusion; sometimes it seems to begin after the patient has begun to show improvement in other respects.

Again, one wonders to what extent delirium tremens might be preventable were each patient who stops abusing alcohol provided with good medical support and pharmacologic treatment for five to seven days following its withdrawal. Certainly the avoidance of delirium tremens is desirable, for it presents a difficult therapeutic problem, response to therapy is often disappointing, its course is sometimes prolonged even with the best treatment, and it is still attended by a significant mortality (see Chap. 3 and Greenblatt and Shader[5]).

DISORDERS DUE TO VITAMIN DEFICIENCY IN CHRONIC ALCOHOLICS

Wernicke-Korsakoff Syndrome[9,10]

The Wernicke-Korsakoff syndrome is a disorder of thiamine deficiency seen most often in chronic alcoholics but also in patients with severe thiamine deficit due to other causes. The onset is usually subacute, its salient features making their appearance over a period of several days to a few weeks.

WERNICKE SYNDROME

The subacute phase, usually called the Wernicke syndrome or Wernicke encephalopathy, is manifested by (1) abnormalities of ocular movement, (2) unsteadiness of station and gait, and (3) changes in mentation. Ocular signs, varying in extent and severity from patient to patient, usually consist of: (1) nystagmus, both horizontal and vertical; (2) weakness or paralysis of the lateral rectus muscles; and (3) weakness or paralysis of conjugate gaze. Internuclear ophthalmoplegia (paralysis of the adducting eye on attempted conjugate lateral gaze, with or without nystagmus in the abducting eye) is common. The pupils are usually normal in size and reactivity. Unsteadiness of station and gait is often severe, and the patient may be unable to stand or walk, but there is often relative sparing of the upper extremities. In the hands and arms, ataxia, past-pointing, and intention tremors may be absent.

Changes in mentation are variable, but a quiet delirium (or as others have called it, a global confusional state) is seen most often. Patients are usually quiet, drowsy, apathetic, inattentive, and indifferent, and, if questioned, they have the global mentative changes characteristic of delirium. Less often patients have the symptoms and signs that commonly attend alcohol withdrawal, but these usually are not severe. Rarely, from the time they are first seen, patients are alert and responsive but have the characteristic features of Korsakoff psychosis (see below).

The symptoms and signs of the Wernicke syndrome can be explained by the lesions found in postmortem examinations in the paraventricular regions of the thalamus and hypothalamus, the mammillary bodies, the periaqueductal region of the midbrain, the floor of the fourth ventricle, and the superior cerebellar vermis. These lesions are specific for thiamine deficiency. Over 80 percent of all patients with the Wernicke syndrome have, in addition, evidence of a peripheral neuropathy. This clinical feature cannot be explained on the basis of thiamine deficiency alone, however, and is thought to be the result of multiple nutritional deficiencies.

Wernicke encephalopathy is a neuropsychiatric emergency; its prompt recognition and immediate treatment is essential if recovery is to occur, and even with the promptest treatment, the results are poor. Every patient suspected of having the Wernicke syndrome should receive 100 mg of thiamine intravenously and 50 mg intramuscularly at once, and 50 mg intramuscularly daily for the next seven days (or until the patient's oral alimentation is again adequate).

The ocular abnormalities are the manifestations of the disorder most responsive to treatment, and often significant improvement is apparent within a matter of hours. Indeed, failure of the ocular abnormalities to improve after treatment with thiamine casts doubt on the diagnosis of the Wernicke syndrome. With time, recovery of eye movements is essentially complete, although patients are often left with some fine nystagmus on lateral gaze. The impairment of station and gait responds slower and less well to treatment. Usually there is slow improvement in the ataxia over one to six weeks, but recovery is incomplete in over one half.

The response of the mentative changes to treatment is the poorest of all. The alcohol withdrawal symptoms usually disappear quickly and cause no serious problems. The symptoms of delirium clear slower, over one to two weeks or sometimes much longer. With the clearing of the global mentative changes of delirium, however, only about 15 to 20 percent of patients with Wernicke encephalopathy regain their premorbid mentative capacities. A large majority is left with the signs and symptoms of the Korsakoff syndrome.

KORSAKOFF SYNDROME

The characteristic clinical features of Korsakoff syndrome or psychosis (also called the amnesic syndrome[13]) may be apparent when the patient is admitted with the neurologic features of the Wernicke syndrome, but more often these features emerge as the delirium begins to clear. The Korsakoff syndrome has the salient feature of a severely disordered memory in a patient in whom other mentative functions and behavior are relatively well preserved.

Victor and associates[9,10] emphasized two major features of this disordered memory: (1) retrograde amnesia, i.e., impaired ability to recall memories that had been well established prior to the onset of the illness, and (2) anterograde amnesia, i.e., impaired ability to lay down new memories for the period following the onset of the illness. In addition to the memory defects, others have considered disorientation and confabulation as essential features of the syndrome.

The retrograde amnesia is neither dense nor complete, but it appears to extend to memories of all periods before the onset of the illness. Talland[6] emphasized that it is not so much the loss of specific memories as it is the inability to put retained memories into proper temporal sequence which gives this retrograde amnesia its particular flavor. Anterograde amnesia is more severe than retrograde amnesia, and in many of these patients there is a virtual inability to lay down new memories after the onset of the illness. The memory defect is thus most apparent and absolute in testing for recent memory. Anterograde amnesia is never absolute, but it may be so severe that the examiner has difficulty finding evidence for new memories laid down after the onset. With such grave defects in recent memory, it is not surprising that disorientation is a regular feature.

Confabulation is striking in many patients, and some observers have considered it a cardinal sign. There is little question, however, that some patients with Korsakoff psychosis do not confabulate. Talland[6] suggested that much which appears to be confabulation may result from the patient's inability to put remote memories into proper temporal sequences. Thus the temporally confused remote memories become a sort of pseudoconfabulation. Victor and associates[9,10] noted that although confabulation may be prominent in the months just after onset, it often disappears in the chronic, plateau phase of the disease.

In addition, Zangwill[13] stressed the striking deficiency of insight in patients with Korsakoff psychosis. They are often unaware that anything is amiss in their lives, or should they possess any awareness, the severity of the defect is minimized or "explained away by facile rationalization." They often appear unconcerned about themselves, and lack of initiative is striking.

The Korsakoff syndrome is as remarkable for those capacities that are preserved as for those that are lost. These patients are alert, aware of their environment, attentive, and articulate. Immediate recall is preserved. They are often able to carry on an animated and appropriate conversation, so long as the topic does not require some specific recent or remote memory. Intellectual capacities are often remarkably well preserved, again so long as memory retrieval is not required to answer the question or solve the problem posed. It can be shown, however, even in situations in which memory retrieval is not the major factor, that these patients' ability to reason and to manipulate ideas is impaired.

The memory defects of the Korsakoff syndrome are the result of the brain lesions due to thiamine deficiency, as described for the Wernicke syndrome. Victor and associates[9,10] emphasized, however, the importance of lesions of the medial dorsal nucleus of the thalamus and perhaps the medial pulvinar in the genesis of the specific memory defects seen in the Korsakoff syndrome.

The phase of Wernicke encephalopathy can be treated with thiamine with expectation for improvement in many of the symptoms and signs, but with the emergence of the signs of the Korsakoff syndrome, there is little that can be done specifically to hasten recovery. Some patients show improvement, often over a period of many months, but only a few recover completely. More patients recover enough that they are able to live with some degree of autonomy; but most are left profoundly and permanently impaired.

Victor and associates[9,10] viewed the Wernicke-Korsakoff syndrome as a single entity; we agree with this viewpoint. The syndrome is specific clinically and pathologically, and its name should be reserved for those patients who fulfill the clinical criteria described in detail above. The name should not be applied indiscriminately to other types of mentative changes associated with alcoholism.

Central Pontine Myelinolysis and Marchiafava-Bignami Disease

Two other neuropathologic entities also are associated with chronic alcoholism—central pontine myelinolysis and Marchiafava-Bignami disease; both are believed to result from nutritional deficiencies. These disorders are rare, however, and it is unlikely that they will be encountered by the practicing psychiatrist.

DEMENTIA IN ALCOHOLICS

Subclinical Deterioration

Chronic ethanol abuse has long been suspected to produce functional and structural cerebral changes aside from those that are the result of chronic nutritional deficits and repeated cerebral trauma. If this be true, one would expect the alcoholic to go through a long period of subclinical deterioration before overt cognitive defects attract attention. The best evidence for this comes from a study by Brewer and Perrett.[1] Using psychologic tests, pneumoencephalograms, and electroencephalograms, they studied a group of male alcoholics and long-term heavy drinkers. None of their patients was over 60, and none had obvious cognitive defects. Most were employed, and they appeared well nourished and well cared for. Nevertheless, 70 percent of their patients had radiologically significant atrophy (cortical sulcal widening being more striking than ventricular enlargement), and, of these, 65 percent had evidence of organic dysfunction on psychologic testing. Earlier Tumarkin and associates[7] had published evidence of cortical and subcortical cerebral atrophy and of psychologic test abnormalities present in a small group of younger subjects who had been drinking excessively for an average period of 11 years. In both these studies, the brain atrophy was attributed to alcohol toxicity per se, not to other factors.

It thus appears likely that chronic alcohol abuse brings about functional and structural changes long before overt cognitive defects appear. It is anticipated that there will soon be a series of well controlled studies using computed cranial tomography to delineate better this period of subclinical brain damage in alcoholics.

Alcoholic Dementia

Alcoholic dementia is a disorder with which most clinicians are familiar but which few have studied or described in detail. Many alcoholics have been observed to experience a chronic dementing illness manifested by cognitive defects in many spheres. The disorder resembles Alzheimer disease much more closely than the Wernicke-Korsakoff syndrome, both in its chronicity and in the global nature of its cognitive defects. Cortical atrophy and ventricular enlargement are frequently demonstrable by radiologic techniques. The course is progressive in those patients who continue to abuse alcohol, but in those who stop drinking there is often slow but significant clinical improvement, even in the presence of significant cerebral atrophy. Dreyfus[3] wrote that in some patients there may be a pattern of stepwise progression, stability or improvement coinciding with sobriety and further worsening following the resumption of drinking.

Regrettably, alcoholic dementia has been the object of few serious studies by either neurologists or psychiatrists. This is perhaps understandable in view of the problems involved in trying to separate patients with this disorder from those with other types of cerebral dysfunction occurring in alcoholics, such as those due to nutritional deficits, trauma, and liver failure. The lack of investigation, is, nevertheless, unfortunate, because there is at least ample anecdotal evidence to suggest that this is one form of dementia which is to some extent specifically treatable—by abstinence from alcohol. One exception to the dearth of investigations is the study of Cutting[2] who showed that patients with alcoholic dementia could be distinguished on clinical grounds from those with the Korsakoff syndrome, although there remained a group of patients in whom features of the two disorders were combined.

We must await further clinical, psychologic, and pathologic studies to gain full understanding of this disorder—if indeed it is a discreet disorder.

REFERENCES

1. Brewer, C., and Perrett, L.: Brain damage due to alcohol consumption: An air-encephalographic, psychometric and electroencephalographic study. Brit. J. Addict. 66:170, 1971.
2. Cutting, J.: The relationship between Korsakov's syndrome and 'alcoholic dementia'. Brit. J. Psychiatry 132:240, 1978.
3. Dreyfus, P.M.: Amblyopia and other neurological disorders associated with chronic alcoholism, in Vinken, P.J., and Bruyn, G.W. (eds.): Handbook of Clinical Neurology, vol. 28. North-Holland Publishing Company, Amsterdam, 1976.
4. Earnest, M.P., and Yarnell, P.R.: Seizure admissions to a city hospital: the role of alcohol. Epilepsia 17:387, 1976.
5. Greenblatt, D.J., and Shader, R.I.: Treatment of the alcohol withdrawal syndrome, in Shader, R.I. (ed.): Manual of Psychiatric Therapeutics. Little Brown and Company, Boston, 1975, pp. 211-235.
6. Talland, G.A.: Deranged Memory: A Psychonomic Study of the Amnesic Syndrome. Academic Press, New York, 1965.
7. Tumarkin, B., Wilson, J.D., and Snyder, G.: Cerebral atrophy due to alcoholism in young adults. U.S. Armed Forces Med. J. 6:67, 1955.
8. Victor, M.: The pathophysiology of alcoholic epilepsy. Res. Publ. Assoc. Res. Nerv. Ment. Dis. 46:431, 1966 (published in 1968).
9. Victor, M.: The Wernicke-Korsakoff Syndrome, in Vinken, P.J., and Bruyn, G.W. (eds.): Handbook of Clinical Neurology, vol. 28. North-Holland Publishing Company, Amsterdam, 1976.
10. Victor, M., Adams, R.D., and Collins, G.H.: The Wernicke-Korsakoff Syndrome. F.A. Davis Company, Philadelphia, 1971.
11. Wikler, A., Pescor, F.T., Fraser, H.F., et al.: Electroencephalographic

changes associated with chronic alcoholic intoxication and the alcohol abstinence syndrome. Am. J. Psychiatry 113:106, 1956.

12. Wolff, H.G., and Curran, D.: Nature of delirium and allied states. Arch. Neurol. Psychiatry 33:1175, 1935.
13. Zangwill, O.L.: The amnesic syndrome, *in* Whitty, C.W.M., and Zangwill, O.L. (eds.): Amnesia, ed. 2. Butterworths, Boston, 1977, pp. 104-117.

CHAPTER 9

CEREBROVASCULAR DISEASE

The psychiatrist seldom is faced with the acute care of a stroke victim. The sudden onset of unilateral weakness or sensory disturbance so universally is recognized as a stroke that the diagnosis usually is made by the patient or family members before seeking medical help. There are, however, several stroke syndromes that do not cause weakness, and these are often misdiagnosed. This is especially likely if symptoms are unusual or bizarre and thus resemble those seen in hysteria or psychosis. Not infrequently psychiatrists are asked to evaluate such patients, and medical colleagues often insist that such patients be accepted for psychiatric care. Psychiatrists also may be asked to consult on other patients who have well recognized stroke syndromes with significant psychiatric sequelae. In this chapter we will review the pathogenesis of cerebrovascular disease, the nonparalytic stroke syndromes, and those aspects of symptomatology and therapy particularly pertinent to the psychiatrist.

In each stroke, there are at least three factors to be considered. First and most basic, the stroke is the result of some type of arterial, or less often venous, disease which results in either occlusion or rupture of the vessel. Second, as a consequence of this, there is brain dysfunction which may be the result of temporary ischemia, ischemic infarction, or hemorrhage. Third and most obvious, there is the abnormal neurologic or behavioral syndrome which is a manifestation of the localized dysfunction or destruction of brain tissue. This abnormality may be the familiar hemiparesis, or it may be a nonparalytic or even primarily behavioral abnormality, particularly if the association areas of the cerebral hemispheres or the cerebellum are the major sites involved. Comprehensive care of the stroke victim rests on the recognition of all three factors and their appropriate management.

PATHOGENESIS

Vascular Diseases

As the term cerebrovascular disease implies, the primary lesion is in the vessels, usually arteries, that supply the brain. These vessels undergo either occlusion, which leads to ischemic infarction of the brain, or rupture, which leads to intracerebral hemorrhage. We will not discuss primary subarachnoid hemorrhage.

THROMBOTIC OCCLUSION

Thrombotic occlusion of an artery seldom occurs de novo but usually requires pre-existing disease. By far the most common intrinsic arterial disease is atherosclerosis; other diseases include arteritis, migraine, meningitis, syphilis, and fibromuscular dysplasia. In all these diseases there is a progressive narrowing of the arterial lumen, and then a thrombus forms in the remaining lumen, thus completing the occlusion.

Atherosclerosis is common in our population and is accelerated by advancing age, hypertension, smoking, diabetes, and hyperlipoproteinemia.[5] The atheromatous plaques tend to occur at predictable sites in the cerebral vasculature. The more common locations are the internal carotid at its origin in the neck and the horizontal stem of the middle cerebral, the vertebral, and the basilar arteries.[12] The atherosclerotic plaque grows, progressively, encroaching upon the arterial lumen. The exposure of subendothelial tissue, especially collagen, to the blood causes platelets and fibrin to accumulate at the site of the plaque.[4] When the luminal diameter has become critically small, a thrombus forms which may complete the occlusion.[1] This process is often referred to as atherothrombosis.

Bits and pieces of this thrombus-laden atherosclerotic plaque may dislodge and be swept distally to occlude smaller intracranial arteries. Because this material is friable, it often fragments so that only transient occlusion occurs. This is the currently postulated pathogenesis of transient ischemic attacks, which occur primarily in the presence of atherosclerotic thrombotic lesions.[7] This is actually an embolic phenomenon, although it is usually treated apart from cerebral embolism as discussed following.

EMBOLIC OCCLUSION[22]

Cerebral arteries free of disease may be occluded by the arrival of an embolus large enough to block the luminal diameter. Emboli are usually fragments of thrombus from the heart or from atheromatous lesions at sites between the heart and the point of occlusion; less often the emboli are composed of air, fat, or tumor. Emboli from the heart are considered to be more common, their formation usually being secondary to underlying cardiac disease such as congenital or rheumatic valve disease, myocardial infarction, endocarditis, or arrhythmias. As mentioned above, emboli from atheromatous lesions may on the one hand cause transient ischemic attacks and on the other cause major strokes.

ARTERIAL RUPTURE

The rupture of small intraparenchymal arteries gives rise to intracerebral hemorrhage. This most often occurs in the setting of longstanding hypertension. The lesion, hypertensive lipohyalinosis, weakens the arterial wall, allowing aneurysmal dilation and rupture. These arteries also may rupture because of trauma, septic embolism, arteritis, arteriovenous malformations, blood dyscrasias, and neoplasms.

BRAIN DISEASES

Ischemia[10] and Infarction

Brain tissue is extremely susceptible to anoxia. Deprivation of blood for 30 seconds disrupts cerebral metabolism and function, and if the anoxia lasts more than 5 minutes, irreversible ischemic infarction occurs. The term stroke connotes the occurrence of circumscribed ischemic infarction of the brain caused by deprivation of oxygenated blood to a specific area. Generalized cerebral ischemia, such as is caused by hypotension and cardiac arrhythmias, produces diffuse cerebral dysfunction. Generally this phenomenon is not termed a stroke.

The size of the cerebral infarct following arterial occlusion depends on the adequacy of collateral blood flow and the relation between the site of occlusion and anastomotic sites. Because these two parameters differ from one patient to another, variation is to be expected in the size of infarcts resulting from arterial occlusions in similar locations in different persons.

Intracerebral Hematoma

Upon rupture of a small penetrating artery, blood extravasates into the brain, disrupting surrounding tissue. The force of the leaking blood may shear other vessels and, in an avalanche fashion, enlarge the hematoma.[11] Brain function is disrupted both by destruction and distortion of usual anatomy. Once the bleeding has ceased, rebleeding usually does not occur.

The size of the extravasations vary from petechial hemorrhages to massive hematomas several centimeters in size. The blood may or may not leak into the ventricular system, but almost never is there leakage through brain directly into the subarachnoid space. The common sites of bleeding, in decreasing order of frequency, are basal ganglia (putamen and caudate nucleus), cerebral white matter, thalamus, pons, and cerebellar hemispheres.

STROKE SYNDROMES

The hallmark of a stroke is the temporal profile of the illness. Regardless of the specific symptoms, the neurologic deficit usually appears rapidly over a period of minutes or hours, rarely a period of days. The nature of the onset depends upon the character of the underlying vascular lesion (see above). In cerebral embolism the onset is usually abrupt, occurring over a period of seconds or a very few minutes, and the deficit is maximum at the onset. The onset of thrombosis is more varied. It is apt to be at night during sleep, and the patient awakens with the symptoms of the stroke. The stroke often progresses in a series of steps, called a stuttering progression, or in a steady progression. Most have reached the maximal neurologic deficit by 48 to 72 hours. Thrombotic strokes are also often preceded by transient cerebral ischemic attacks, which are shorter (less than 24 hours) versions of the stroke to come. Cerebral hemorrhages usually occur over a period of minutes to hours of smooth progression, accompanied by headache, nausea, and vomiting.

Improvement is the rule in all who survive strokes; it may begin almost immediately, as in transient ischemic attacks and cerebral embolism, or within the first week or so. Occasionally, there is temporary worsening caused by edema around the brain lesion.

The specific symptoms of a stroke depend on which cerebral vessel is affected and in turn on which area of the brain is involved. We will not discuss in detail the more common neurovascular syndromes which seldom cause confusion in diagnosis, but we will attend more fully to the nonparalytic stroke syndromes. Occlusion of the internal carotid artery often is asymptomatic if there is adequate collateral circulation, but it may cause symptoms of ipsilateral monocular blindness, contralateral hemiparesis and hemianesthesia, aphasia if the dominant hemisphere is involved, and even less often homonymous hemianopsia. Occlusion of the anterior cerebral artery is recognized by the predominance of the motor and sensory symptoms in the contralateral foot and leg. The syndrome of middle cerebral artery occlusion is similar to internal carotid occlusion except that the eye is spared, homonymous hemianopsia is more common, and the hemiparesis is often more pronounced. Occlusion in the vertebrobasilar system usually combines unilateral or bilateral motor and sensory deficits involving the extremities with obvious brain stem dysfunction, e.g., diplopia, ataxia, crossed motor and sensory signs, dysarthia, dysphagia, or dysfunction of cranial nerves III through XII.

Nonparalytic Stroke Syndromes

We will now consider the more obscure stroke syndromes which might be encountered by the psychiatrist and present some trouble in accurate diagnosis. The syndromes that occur in the various arterial territories will be discussed.

CAROTID ARTERIAL SYSTEM

OPHTHALMIC ARTERY. This is the first major branch of the internal carotid artery. Its branch, the central retinal artery, supplies the optic nerve and retina. Either the ophthalmic or the central retinal artery may be involved, either by intrinsic disease or by emboli from a more proximal source. Two major syndromes are related to occlusion of this artery.

Amaurosis fugax is a transient monocular blindness which is brief in duration (usually 1 to 15 minutes) and rarely exceeds 30 minutes. It begins with a black or gray shade or curtain smoothly descending or ascending within 1 or 2 seconds to obscure all or part of monocular vision. At times a fog or blur is described. Vision is fully restored.

Because the episodes of blindness are so brief, the physician rarely has the opportunity to examine the symptomatic patient. In an examination during the attack, Fisher[8] noted white plugs, thought to be platelet-fibrin masses, coursing through the retinal arteries. The diagnosis is made primarily on the basis of historical data. Approximately 50 to 60 percent are associated with internal carotid occlusive disease. Other causes include cranial arteritis, migraine, papilledema, global retinal ischemia, and oral contraceptive pills.

Permanent monocular blindness usually occurs suddenly. The etiology is presumed to be an occlusion of the ophthalmic or central retinal artery. Often the cause is not apparent after arteriography. Extracranial vascular disease and aortic valvular disease must be considered as sources of embolism.

ANTERIOR CEREBRAL ARTERY. Specific syndromes of the anterior cerebral artery have been imperfectly studied. Only when motor or sensory symptoms predominately involve the foot and leg can the diagnosis of isolated anterior cerebral artery disease comfortably be made. Branches of the proximal portion of the anterior cerebral artery pierce the substance and supply the white matter beneath the frontal lobe cortex. It is possible, therefore, that infarction of the white matter beneath Broca's speech area in the frontal lobe could produce an isolated

147

aphasia syndrome resembling that due to infarction of Broca's area. It is also possible that infarction of the frontal poles could result in an isolated frontal lobe syndrome. Neither of these is, however, a usual sequel to anterior cerebral artery occlusion.

MIDDLE CEREBRAL ARTERY. Oftentimes isolated aphasic syndromes are caused by occlusions of cortical branches of the middle cerebral artery with resulting circumscribed infarctions of the dominant cerebral hemisphere. Typically, there is the sudden onset of fluent, paraphasic speech and impaired auditory comprehension characteristic of Wernicke's aphasia (see Chap. 2). Conduction aphasia, Broca's aphasia, and Gerstman's syndrome are encountered less often. When the onset is acute, these syndromes should be attributed to a stroke. The most likely etiology is embolism to the smaller middle cerebral artery branches.

Less frequently recognized than isolated aphasia syndromes are isolated nondominant hemisphere syndromes. These occur with occlusions of branches of the middle cerebral artery in the nondominant hemisphere. Symptoms vary considerably but most often consist of clumsiness of the left hand, dressing or constructional apraxia, and inattention to and denial of the left side of space.

POSTERIOR CEREBRAL ARTERY. Syndromes of posterior cerebral artery strokes may be divided into proximal and distal, depending on which of the areas supplied by the artery are involved. The distal portion of the posterior cerebral artery supplies the medial temporal and occipital lobes. From the proximal segment of this artery arise penetrating branches which pierce through the posterior perforating substance and supply blood to the thalamus, hypothalamus and subthalamus.

The major proximal artery syndrome is the pure sensory stroke.[9] This is caused by a small infarct (lacunar infarction) in the central sensory relay nuclei of the thalamus. These patients complain of subjective sensory symptoms on the opposite side of the body which split the midline, and on examination one finds decreased sensation to multiple sensory modalities corresponding to the symptomatic areas.

At times this pattern of sensory loss may be difficult to distinguish from conversion symptoms. In the pure sensory stroke, the patients seldom complain of other symptoms such as weakness, pain, or visual disturbance. Although total loss of sensation seldom occurs, Fisher[9] mentioned that the sensory symptoms usually so overshadow the physical finding that the syndrome might be called the pure paresthetic stroke. In the hemisensory loss of a conversion reaction, we have found it useful to test vibratory sense over the forehead and nose. Since these boney structures are essentially fused to make one large bone, the vibratory sense should not change abruptly near the midline as does the ability to appreciate pain or touch.

A small infarct or hemorrhage in the subthalamic nucleus causes hemiballismus—a wild, flinging, uncontrollable movement in the contralateral limbs. Choreiform and athetoid movements on one side of the body may also result from infarcts in this area.

Most distal artery syndromes include as at least part of the symptomatology a contralateral homonymous hemianopsia, because the primary visual area, the calcarine cortex of the occipital lobe, is at the distal end of the posterior cerebral artery. Most of the time this is the only finding. Other symptoms and signs of distal artery syndromes are built upon a homonymous hemianopsia, depending upon what additional ischemic damage is done and its location.

When the infarction involves the left medial occipital lobe and the splenium of the corpus callosum, the patient develops a right hemianopsia and the syndrome of alexia without agraphia.[18] These patients can speak and write fluently without mistakes, but they cannot read aloud what they have just written. Other accompanying symptoms may be color dysnomia and disturbances of recent memory.[21] Possibly a variation of this is the syndrome of agitated delirium with visual impairment.[20] This syndrome occurs in the presence of either hemianopsia or bilateral cortical blindness. Patients usually have the onset of visual impairment followed within hours or a couple of days by an agitated delirium. The patient may not be aware of the visual deficit. When the delirium clears, the visual impairment and short-term memory deficit often persist, although other cortical functions may be left intact. On computed cranial tomography the lesion involves one or both medial temporal and occipital lobes.

Memory disturbances are frequent in patients with posterior cerebral artery occlusion. Ischemic damage to the inferior medial temporal lobe, including the hippocampus, is thought to cause this disturbance. Generally it has been considered necessary to have bilateral temporal lobe lesions in order to disrupt memory, but there have been many instances of amnesia following unilateral, usually dominant, temporal lobe infarcts.[3,21] The amnesia of unilateral temporal lobe damage may improve with time in contrast to that seen in bilateral damage. It is important to realize that the amnesia does not occur alone but is accompanied by other evidence of neurologic dysfunction in the territory of the posterior cerebral artery, e.g., homonymous hemianopsia and alexia without agraphia.

A peculiar amnestic anomia may be seen with dominant temporal lobe lesions.[2] These patients usually are alert and display good auditory and visual comprehension, but they are unable to use nouns in spontaneous speech or to name objects presented visually. They are able to demonstrate the use for the object, identify it from a group when given the name, and speak the name on repetition tasks. Other tasks of memory are performed well. There may be a homonymous visual field deficit, especially a homonymous upper quadranopsia, because of involvement of that part of the visual radiation which courses through the temporal lobe. Abscess, localized encephalitis (herpes simplex), tumor, hemorrhage, and infarction have all been found to cause this syndrome.

Cerebrovascular disease is often regarded as the cause of the syndrome of transient global amnesia (see Chap. 13). However, the lack of other neurologic symptoms and signs and of good pathologic evidence makes ready acceptance of this theory difficult.

VERTEBROBASILAR ARTERY

The major syndrome of vertebral artery occlusion is the Wallenberg or lateral medullary syndrome.[14] The occlusion occurs at the site of origin of the posterior inferior cerebellar artery and blocks both the vertebral and the posterior inferior cerebellar arteries. Less often, this syndrome is caused by occlusion of the posterior inferior cerebellar artery alone. The infarction lies in the posterolateral aspect of the medulla, sparing the more anterior corticospinal tracts (and thus producing no paralysis). The symptoms and signs include impairment of pain and thermal sense over the contralateral arm and leg and sometimes over the face ipsilaterally, ipsilateral Horner's syndrome, hoarseness, dysphagia, dysarthia, vertigo, nausea, ipsilaterally diminished gag reflex, and ipsilateral ataxia.

Occlusion of the basilar artery usually causes a catastrophic stroke with coma or at least bilateral paralysis. Oftentimes the smaller branches of the basilar artery which penetrate into the pons may occlude causing limited syndromes. These, termed basilar branch syndromes,[13] cause various combinations of brain stem deficits.

The cerebellum is supplied by three major arteries, and occlusion of any of them may cause infarction. Likewise, hemorrhage into the cerebellum may occur. Both of these conditions are important because of the potentially disastrous results if swelling takes place and causes significant brain stem compression. Cerebellar hemorrhage[15] evolves over several hours. Usually there is sudden onset of dizziness with headache, vomiting, and severe imbalance, preventing even standing. Downward pressure on the pons may cause ipsilateral VI or VII cranial nerve palsies or a conjugate lateral gaze palsy. Weakness of the extremities usually does not occur until late when coma sets in.

Cerebellar infarction may go unrecognized or cause little difficulty unless the postinfarction edema creates a mass effect and compresses the vital centers of the brain stem. The early symptoms[6] which have received little attention include the sudden onset of rotatory dizziness, nausea, vomiting, horizontal nystagmus, and imbalance. The syndrome of cerebellar infarction closely resembles that of a nonspecific labyrinthine disorder.

PSYCHIATRIC SEQUELAE AND MANAGEMENT IN STROKE

The psychiatrist who sees a stroke patient because of behavioral distur- bances can usually be sure that the etiology of the behavioral difficulties is mutifactoral, i.e., a mixture of organic and psychologic determinants. The fact that strokes usually afflict older adults, the disturbance in normal behavior caused by cerebral damage, and the patient's reactions to the neurologic deficit all play important etiologic roles.

The organic determinants of the behavioral disturbances are of prime importance, but a narrow focusing on organic features should not be allowed to lead to neglect of psychologic components. The nature and severity of the organically based changes depend on both the site and size of infarcted brain tissue. Even a small lesion that results in unyield- ing hemiplegia may result in profound behavioral consequences, but in this instance the behavioral consequences probably result more from the psychologic reaction to the disability than from the cognitive loss. Even a small lesion that results in severe aphasia will probably effect significant behavioral changes, but in this instance it is likely to be a result of both the cognitive loss and the frustration resulting from the loss. If we look at cognitive changes per se, however, the extent of cognitive loss is related closely to the mass of brain tissue infarcted.[24] Except when such vital areas as speech centers are involved, cognitive changes are seldom noticeable when 50 ml or less of brain tissue is lost through infarction. Measurable cognitive loss increases progressively, however, with infarction of larger and larger amounts of brain sub- stance.

In discussing the cognitive loss resulting from strokes, it should be emphasized once more that strokes are not often the cause of the slowly progressive dementias.[25] When profound cognitive loss results from multiple small strokes, there is almost always a history of acute exacer- bations followed by some degree of remission, focal neurologic symptoms or signs, and/or long-standing hypertension.

Another behavioral consequence of strokes, denial of illness, also may be the result of organic and/or psychologic factors. One type of denial of illness, anosognosia, is seen most often in nondominant hemispheric strokes (especially those involving the parietal lobe) and is thought to be a feature of the anatomic site of the damage. In this situation, there is an indifference to or an unawareness of the hemiplegia, and the patient acts as if nothing happened. In its most severe form, the patient, when shown the paralyzed arm, denies ownership, going so far in some in- stances as to suggest that it is an artificial limb or that it belongs to another patient. Usually anosognosia is associated with sensory and visual disturbances as well as with decreased attentiveness, mild confu- sion, and lethargy. Another organically determined type of denial of illness is that seen in patients with moderate to severe degrees of diffuse cerebral hemisphere damage. This too is primarily an unawareness of the presence of defects and limitations. It is seen more often in patients with diffuse degenerative neurologic diseases than with strokes, but it may be seen when multiple small infarcts cause diffuse brain dysfunction.

Psychologically determined denial of illness also occurs in stroke victims, but there is no evidence that this specific type of denial occurs any more frequently in patients with organic brain lesions than with other somatic diseases. This type of denial is marked not so much by a failure of recognition of neurologic defects as by a denial of their consequences. Thus a patient may discuss intelligently the existence of a hemiparesis but at the same time insist that this will not significantly impair his or her usual motor activities. In large part, this reaction to illness appears to be based on premorbid personality; it occurs especially in patients whose previous lives were marked by conspicuous, exaggerated traits of independence, traits which probably concealed fears of dependency along with excessive dependency needs. This type of reaction is unrelated to site or extent of brain damage.

Depression, common in stroke patients, usually has been attributed to the severity of the neurologic disability and to the sudden deterioration of life patterns and potentials. Post[23] noted, however, that depressive illnesses were more common in stroke patients than in others, and Folstein and coworkers,[17] in a comparison between stroke patients and equally disabled orthopaedic patients, found depression significantly more often among the stroke victims (45 percent versus 10 percent). In addition, these workers found a constellation of symptoms (including subjective irritability, loss of interest, poor concentration, subjective memory difficulty, and anhedonia) much more frequently in patients with right hemisphere (nondominant) strokes than in those with left hemisphere strokes or orthopaedic disabilities. These latter observations recall those of Flor-Henry,[16] who found that epilepsy involving the nondominant temporal lobe often was associated with symptoms which suggested manic-depressive disease. Folstein and associates[17] suggested that mood disorder is a specific symptom of stroke and not a psychologic reaction to the disability.

Other psychologic reactions to stroke may be encountered. Anxiety is common, because of fear both of the consequences of the stroke and of further strokes. Anxiety, if not completely disabling, can be a stimulus for a realistic approach to the new situation. Anger too may be a problem. It is more often seen in younger patients, especially when there is disabling paralysis in the presence of preserved intellect. Severe psychologic regression is not seen as often as one might expect in light of the severe incapacity which often occurs, but profound dependency develops in some patients.

Specific management of these psychological sequelae of strokes is difficult. For most of these patients, it is wise to follow the advice that Lewis[19] gave for patients with post-traumatic syndromes, i.e., not to insist upon answering with any finality the question if the symptoms are due to structural damage or to psychologic influences. Most of the time a mixture of organic and emotional features will be at play and they must be dealt with concurrently. We have found that repeated explanations of the illness, competent and understanding rehabilitation, and consistent family support are the more potent therapeutic agents. Anxiety can be transformed into a positive stimulus through the offer of insight and hope of recovery. Anger is more difficult to deal with, but a consistent, firm, understanding, and affectually neutral stance is most therapeutic. However, both anxiety and anger may be of such intensity that they seriously interfere with medical care and rehabilitation. When this is the case, the anxiolytic agents may be valuable, treatment with them (as with all neuroleptics) starting with doses lower than would be used in patients without brain damage. Occasionally the antipsychotic agents are prescribed, especially in the presence of overwhelming anxiety or paranoid ideation.

Although depression is often severe, suicide fortunately is uncommon. The studies of both Post[23] and Folstein and associates[17] suggest a special relationship between strokes and depression, but they do not imply that depression should be accepted as a necessary consequence of cerebrovascular accidents. The depression which follows stroke should be treated like any other, with supportive psychotherapy and antidepressant medications. The patient's cardiovascular status and compromised cerebral function may require special caution both as to the choice of antidepressant and as to dosage, but the response to treatment is often gratifying.

REFERENCES

1. Adams, R.D., and Fisher, C.M.: Pathology of cerebral arterial occlusion, *in* Fields, W.S. (ed.): Pathogenesis and Treatment of Cerebrovascular Disease. Charles C Thomas, Springfield, Ill., 1961.
2. Adams, R.D., and Mohr, J.P.: Affections of speech, *in* Wintrobe, M.M., et al. (eds.): Harrison's Principles of Internal Medicine, ed. 7. McGraw-Hill Book Company, New York, 1974.
3. Benson, F., Marsden, C.D., and Meadows, J.C.: The amnestic syndrome of posterior cerebral artery occlusion. Acta Neurol. Scand. 50:133, 1974.
4. Deykin, D.: Thrombogenesis. New Engl. J. Med. 276:622, 1967.
5. Duncan, G.W., Lees, R.D., Ojemann, R.G., et al.: Concomitants of atherosclerotic carotid artery stenosis. Stroke 8:665, 1977.
6. Duncan, G.W., Parker, S.W., and Fisher, C.M.: Acute cerebellar infarction in PICA territory. Arch. Neurol. 32:364, 1975.
7. Duncan, G.W., Pessin, M., Mohr, J.P., et al.: Transient cerebral ischemic attacks, *in* Stollerman, G.H. (ed.): Advances in Internal Medicine, Vol. 21. Year Book Medical Publishers, Chicago, 1976.

8. Fisher, C.M.: Observations of the fundus oculi in transient monocular blindness. Neurology 9:337, 1959.
9. Fisher, C.M.: Pure sensory stroke involving face, arm, and leg. Neurology 15:76, 1965.
10. Fisher, C.M.: Cerebral ischemia—less familiar types, in Keener, E.B. (ed.): Clinical Neurosurgery, Vol. 18. Williams and Wilkins, Baltimore, 1971.
11. Fisher, C.M.: Pathological observations in hypertensive cerebral hemorrhage. J. Neuropathol. Exp. Neurol. 30:536, 1971.
12. Fisher, C.M.: The anatomy and pathology of the cerebral vasculature, in Meyer, J.S. (ed.): Modern Concepts of Cerebrovascular Disease. Spectrum Publications, New York, 1975.
13. Fisher, C.M., and Caplan, L.R.: Basilar artery branch occlusion: A cause of pontine infarction. Neurology 21:900, 1971.
14. Fisher, C.M., Karnes, W.E., and Kubik, C.S.: Lateral medullary infarction—the pattern of vascular occlusion. J. Neuropathol. Exp. Neurol. 20:323, 1961.
15. Fisher, C.M., Picard, E.H., Pollak, A., et al.: Acute hypertensive cerebellar hemorrhage: Diagnosis and surgical treatment. J. Nerv. Ment. Dis. 140:38, 1965.
16. Flor-Henry, P.: Psychosis and temporal lobe epilepsy. A controlled investigation. Epilepsia 10:363, 1969.
17. Folstein, M.F., Maiberger, R., and McHugh, P.R.: Mood disorder as a specific complication of stroke. J. Neurol. Neurosurg. Psychiatry 40:1018, 1977.
18. Geschwind, N.: Disconnection syndromes in animals and man. Brain 88:237, 1965.
19. Lewis, A.: Discussion on differential diagnosis and treatment of post-contusional states. Proc. Roy. Soc. Med. 35:607, 1942.
20. Medina, J.L., Chokroverty, S., and Rubin, F.A.: Syndrome of agitated delirium and visual impairment: A manifestation of medial temporo-occipital infarction. J. Neurol. Neurosurg. Psychiatry 40:861, 1977.
21. Mohr, J.P., Leicester, J., Stoddard, L.T., et al.: Right hemianopia with memory and color deficits in circumscribed left posterior artery territory infarction. Neurology 21:1104, 1971.
22. McDowell, F.H.: Cerebral embolism, in Vinken, G.W., and Bruyn, G.W. (eds.): Handbook of Clinical Neurology, Vol. 11. North-Holland Publishing Company, Amsterdam, 1972.
23. Post, F.: Dementia, depression, and pseudodementia, in Benson, D.F., and Blumer, D. (eds.): Psychiatric Aspects of Neurologic Disease. Grune and Stratton, New York, 1975.
24. Tomlinson, B.E.: The pathology of dementia, in Wells, C.E. (ed.): Dementia, ed. 2. F.A. Davis Company, Philadelphia, 1977.
25. Wells, C.E.: Role of stroke in dementia. Stroke 9:1, 1978.

CHAPTER 10

SYNCOPE AND DIZZINESS

Syncope and dizziness are common symptoms that are often difficult to differentiate from one another on the basis of history, usually because patients are unable to describe the symptoms to physicians in terms that have precise and specific meaning. As with headaches, the physician should not accept the patient's complaint at face value but must inquire about the exact nature of the sensation experienced. Often this necessitates resorting to direct and leading questions or ascertaining if the symptoms are similar to those experienced occasionally by most of us, e.g., like "when you stand quickly from a stooped position" or "the feeling after being whirled around on a merry-go-round." A clear definition of the symptom is a prerequisite for establishing the etiology.

SYNCOPE

Seldom does the patient name the symptom as syncope; terms such as blackout, faint, dropout, or weak spells are usually used. In general the physician recognizes two states: (1) syncope, which means complete loss of consciousness and (2) faintness or near-faint, which is that part of a syncopal attack prior to complete loss of consciousness, i.e., the prodrome.

Symptom Analysis

The patient usually describes a sense of feeling unwell along with sensations of nausea (sometimes with vomiting), dizziness, generalized weakness, fading of sight and hearing so that objects and sounds seem to be distant, and pounding and ringing in the head. Observers often describe pallor of the face and profuse perspiration. If the attack proceeds no further, it is termed faintness or near-faint, but if unconsciousness occurs, the term syncope or syncopal attack is used. Unconsciousness usually lasts for only a few seconds, rarely for a full minute. Consciousness is regained more quickly if the patient falls or is placed in a recumbent position. Once the patient begins to awaken, it is accomplished quickly, and the patient feels well almost immediately.

If unconsciousness lasts more than a few seconds, particularly if an upright position is maintained, convulsive or myoclonic movements may occur, but a full-blown tonic-clonic generalized convulsion is rare. At times it may be difficult to distinguish syncope from an epileptic seizure. A seizure usually comes on quicker (without the prodrome of faintness that characterizes syncope), may occur at any time or in any position (often even while asleep), may have focal movements at the outset, is often accompanied by tongue biting and incontinence, usually has a more symptomatic and prolonged postictal stage, and frequently is associated with an abnormal interictal electroencephalogram. Even with all these potentially distinguishing features, the differentiation is often difficult, and the physician may have to resort to therapeutic trials of anticonvulsants in the effort to establish a diagnosis.

Etiology

In general, faintness and syncope are the result of transient inadequacy of total cerebral oxygenation or nutrition. The inadequacy is most frequently the result of insufficient blood flow to the brain, less frequently of too little oxygen or glucose in the blood supplied. Syncope is seldom caused by a localized deficiency in cerebral blood flow as is the case in stroke. Psychiatric disorders also often produce similar symptoms.

Failure of blood to reach the brain in adequate amounts may be the result of (1) failure of the heart to pump enough blood to keep the brain perfused or (2) failure to maintain adequate arterial blood pressure or blood volume.

REDUCED CARDIAC OUTPUT

For several reasons, the heart may fail to pump sufficient amounts of blood to the brain. The myocardial pumping action may be inadequate because of myocardial infarction or myocardiopathy of various types. Arrhythmias may cause syncope, either by reducing the heart rate below 30 to 35 beats per minute or by increasing it to above 150 or so. Patients with complete heart block develop a ventricular rate of approximately 40 or less per minute, but this does not necessarily cause either faintness or syncope. If the block is intermittent, however, a sudden reduction of heart rate often leads to syncope; and if the ventricular rate slows below 30 to 35 beats or if asystole of several seconds duration occurs, faintness or syncope is likely. Stenosis of the aortic valve or the subaortic area may obstruct flow out of the left ventricle to the brain. On the other hand, a reduction in the amount of blood returned to the heart will result in inadequate cardiac output and thus inadequate cerebral blood flow; this condition can be created by the Valsalva maneuver with such acts as coughing, sneezing, straining at stool or micturition, and lifting.

REDUCED BLOOD PRESSURE

Adequate blood pressure depends on maintenance of proper arterial tone (peripheral arterial resistance) and cardiac output. When the normal person stands up from a sitting or supine position, the sympathetic nervous system, triggered by baroreceptors, responds to maintain arterial blood pressure, increasing peripheral resistance by peripheral vasoconstriction and increased cardiac rate and force of contraction. Intermittent, transitory drops in arterial blood pressure in the presence of an adequate cardiac output are usually the result of disordered vasomotor reflexes. Orthostatic hypotension results from inadequate vasomotor reflexes. On standing, blood pressure, and in turn cerebral perfusion, drops, and faintness or syncope ensues. Some of the diseases and conditions which predispose to faulty vasomotor reflexes are peripheral neuropathies (especially when autonomic nerves are involved), spinal cord lesions, the Shy-Drager syndrome, old age, prolonged bed rest, familial dysautonomia, and medications (e.g., antihypertensives, levodopa, antidepressants).

Vasovagal (vasodepressor) syncope is the most common type of faintness and syncope. Engel[3] has elucidated its pathogenesis. There is combined excessive peripheral vasodilation and vagal discharge, so that adequate blood pressure cannot be maintained. The stimulus for vasodilation either overpowers the sympathetic vasoconstrictor response or occurs in a setting of faulty vasomotor reflex activity as discussed above. The vasodilatation occurs first and lowers blood pressure; then, in addition, vagal stimulation slows the heart instead of allowing an increase in the heart rate to help maintain blood pressure. Engel postulated that vasodepressor syncope is a consequence of experiencing fear of injury (actual, threatened, or imagined) and of the inability to react to it. Excessive vasodilation occurs also with pain, strong emotions, medication, alcohol, and overeating.

IMPAIRED CEREBRAL NUTRITION

Too little blood or too little glucose or oxygen in the blood also may cause episodic symptoms of faintness and, if severe, even loss of consciousness or profound coma (see Chaps. 3 and 4). When blood loss is obvious, the differential diagnosis of syncope is not germane. However, blood loss that is not apparent (usually into the gastrointestinal tract) may impair the ability to maintain blood pressure, especially with postural changes, and result in faintness or syncope. A reflex tachycardia accompanying orthostatic hypotension is a clue to the hypovolemia. Demonstration of blood in the stool or of anemia helps establish the diagnosis. Other causes of hypovolemia include Addison disease, dehydration, and prolonged bed rest.

Hypoglycemia causes faintness and syncope because the brain is insufficiently supplied with the essential substrate for its metabolism. Episodic hypoglycemia, which might be described by symptoms of faintness or syncope, may be caused by reactive hypoglycemia, pancreatic tumors (islets of Langerhans), or severe liver disease. With hypoglycemia, the onset of symptoms is usually less abrupt and their progression more gradual than with faintness and syncope due to cardiovascular dysfunction.

PSYCHIATRIC DISORDERS

Psychiatric disorders may be associated with symptoms that resemble both faintness and syncope. Probably the most common cause is anxiety, especially when the anxiety is associated with changes in autonomic nervous system activity (with or without actual compromise in cerebral blood flow). In addition, anxiety often provokes hyperventilation, causing hypocarbia and, in turn, reduced cerebral perfusion. Indeed, hyperventilation is one of the most common causes of faintness, and even syncope may be seen with extremely prolonged hyperventilation.

Hysteria is said to be the second most common cause of episodes that resemble syncope, only vasovagal syncope exceeds it in frequency. As with other hysterical symptoms, it occurs more often in women, and other conversion symptoms often have recurred since adolescence. The unconcerned attitude, *la belle indifference,* is a feature that suggests hysteria, but worry and fear about the symptoms probably are encountered more frequently. Syncope as a conversion reaction usually occurs in the presence of witnesses, and the symptoms are dramatic in their presentation and often sexually suggestive. Personal injury is rare. The autonomic disturbances that are seen in true syncope are absent. Nevertheless, the distinction between syncope as a conversion reaction and syncope of organic etiology may be difficult.

DIZZINESS

Dizziness is a symptom encountered in the patients of virtually all physicians whatever their specialty. It is a subjective, personal sensation, difficult to describe clearly to another person, meaning different things to different people, and usually referring to an unpleasant cephalic sensation of some sort. Strict adherence to the standard clinical methods of gathering information from a thorough history and careful examination will establish the cause of the dizziness in most instances.

158

Symptom Analysis

First the physician must define the meaning to be conveyed in the patient's choice of the word dizziness. Drachman[1] suggested that most patients choose the complaint of dizziness to refer to one of four sensations: (1) an awareness of an impending faint; (2) a definite sensation of rotation (vertigo) or of spatial imbalance; (3) a sense of dysequilibrium present on walking; (4) an imprecise feeling best conveyed by the words "lightheadedness" or "giddiness." Also, the complaint of dizziness sometimes refers to other discrete symptoms such as weakness or visual blurring. However, even most careful and persistent questioning sometimes fails to clarify the complaint. In these instances, the precise nature of the complaint can often be established if the symptom can be precipitated during the clinical examination.

Drachman and Hart[2] suggested several maneuvers that might be used to precipitate the symptom; sudden rising from supine to standing posture (with blood pressure determinations lying, standing, and after standing for 3 minutes); the Valsalva maneuver; carotid sinus stimulation; hyperventilation for 3 minutes; rotation of the head to left and then to right for 15 seconds as if watching a plane; the Nylen-Bárány maneuver (Fig. 10-1); rotating the patient 10 times in 20 seconds (the standard Bárány test); having the patient take a sudden turn while walking. After each maneuver the patient is asked if dizziness occurred, and if so, whether this sensation of dizziness matched the presenting complaint.

The first five maneuvers are designed to create changes in cerebral perfusion which most often would create sensations of faintness but

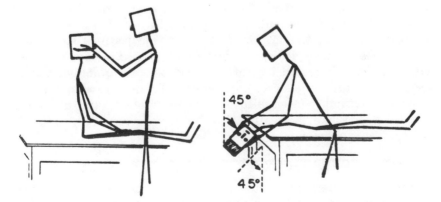

FIGURE 10-1. The Nylen-Bárány maneuver. The patient is moved abruptly from a sitting posture to a supine position with the head held 45° backward and below the plane of the body and tilted 45° to one side. The patient is observed for the appearance of vertigo and nystagmus. The test is then repeated with the head tilted toward the opposite side. (Reproduced from Drachman, D.A. and Hart, C.W.[2] with permission.)

159

might also cause vertigo; the Nylen-Bárány and Bárány tests are used to precipitate vertigo; and the sudden turn, a sense of dysequilibrium. The precise delineation of the symptom is important for the direction that it provides the physician in the quest for the etiology of the dizziness. Thus, a sense of faintness most often signals a sudden reduction in cerebral metabolism due to systemic disease; vertigo and spatial imbalance are most often due to neurologic or otologic disease; dysequilibrium on walking, usually the result of neurologic disease; and lightheadedness, most often associated with psychiatric disorders.

In addition to the specific character of the symptom, the physician in evaluating the history pays especial attention to the patient's age, the abruptness and duration of the attacks, the persistence or intermittency of the symptoms, and the relationship of the symptoms to position or motion. All these features may aid in establishing disease diagnosis, but often extensive general medical, neurologic, otologic, and psychiatric evaluations are required before exact disease diagnosis can be established.

Etiology

The causes of dizziness can best be discussed under the headings of systemic, neurologic, otologic, and psychiatric disorders.

SYSTEMIC DISORDERS

Systemic disorders usually cause dizziness because of reduced cerebral perfusion, thus creating symptoms of faintness and impending syncope. Probably the most common systemic disorder causing dizziness is orthostatic hypotension. The systemic blood pressure falls when the erect position is assumed secondary to (1) poor autonomic reflexes as occurs in peripheral neuropathies, spinal cord lesions, Shy-Drager syndrome, old age, familial dysautonomia, and toxicity from medications (e.g., antihypertensives, levodopa, antidepressants); (2) reduced plasma volume as seen in Addison disease, dehydration, blood loss, and prolonged bed rest; and (3) idiopathic orthostatic hypotension. Primary cardiac disorders such as arrhythmias, heart failure, and outflow obstruction also reduce cerebral blood flow episodically. This topic was covered fully in the first section of this chapter.

NEUROLOGIC DISORDERS

Neurologic disorders most often produce the varieties of dizziness described as vertigo or spatial imbalance and movement dysequilibrium, but some localized vascular disorders affecting the brain and brain stem occasionally cause sensations of faintness as well. Although the sensation of turning or spinning (vertigo) is most specific for involvement of

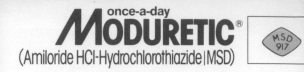

once-a-day
MODURETIC®
(Amiloride HCl-Hydrochlorothiazide | MSD)

MSD
917

MSD
MERCK
SHARP &
DOHME

Before prescribing, please s
Prescribing Information on last pag

7-82   L0792-11,1282-3385   PRINTED IN U.S

the vestibular pathways by either neurologic or otologic disease, the physician should not insist that the symptom conform to true vertigo before considering a disorder affecting the vestibular connections. There are numerous instances of peripheral and central vestibular disorders producing a nonspinning dizziness best described as a sense of spatial imbalance.

The neurologic illnesses that cause vertigo and spatial imbalance usually are disorders that affect the vestibular nerve or vestibular nuclei in the brain stem. Rarely, dysfunction in other parts of the nervous system causes dizziness—for example, in seizures of temporal lobe origin the aura may be dizziness, either spinning or nonspinning. However, it would be most unusual for this symptom to occur alone, in the absence of other manifestations of epilepsy.

Diseases of the brain stem commonly produce dizziness because of the proximity of the vestibular nuclei and their peripheral and central connections. This type can be readily recognized when accompanied by other brain stem symptoms such as nystagmus, diplopia, dysarthria, dysphagia, and ataxia. Dizziness may result from any brain stem disorder, including tumors and multiple sclerosis, but the most common cause is insufficiency of the vertebrobasilar vascular system.

Fisher[4] carefully analyzed the frequency and types of dizziness that occur in ischemic syndromes of the various cerebral arteries. Whereas dizziness occurred in none of the anterior cerebral artery cases and in only 8 percent of internal carotid-middle cerebral artery and 24 percent of posterior cerebral artery cases, it was present in 77 percent of the basilar artery cases. The dizziness was a symptom both of the preceding transient ischemic attacks and of the stroke itself. Because of this, when middle-aged and elderly subjects are seen because of the recent onset of transient dizziness, the possibility of vertebrobasilar insufficiency must be considered. Nevertheless, Fisher found that in most instances the dizziness did not occur as an isolated symptom but was accompanied by dysarthria, facial numbness, hemiparesis, headache, diplopia, or other evidence of brain stem dysfunction. He stated that if dizziness had recurred for more than six weeks without other brain stem symptoms, the etiology was most likely not vertebrobasilar insufficiency.

Dizziness described as a dysequilibrium present chiefly when maintaining an erect posture, walking, or turning is usually associated with overt and relatively severe neurologic disease. It is generally most conspicuous with frontal lobe disease that produces an apraxia of gait and with Parkinson disease. Strokes of the cerebellum without brain stem involvement also may be responsible. In addition, this type of dysequilibrium is ascribed to multiple sensory deficits. For example, loss of vision causes spatial disorientation, and if there is additional sensory loss, such as that due to peripheral neuropathy, the deficits appear to be cumulative in their causation of dysequilibrium. This was one of the more common causes of dizziness found in Drachman and Hart's large group of patients with a primary complaint of dizziness.[2] It has been suggested that disorders of the cervical spine and surrounding musculature, through their connections with the vestibular nuclei, cause dizziness, but this has not been firmly established.

Rarely, the dysequilibrium associated with apraxia of gait may be confused with the dizziness that is sometimes a complaint in hysterical astasia-abasia. Astasia-abasia is usually differentiated from apraxia of gait by the absence of other evidence of neurologic dysfunction and sometimes by the ability of the patient with astasia-abasia to walk normally in certain situations (e.g., at home but not outside).

OTOLOGIC DISORDERS

Otologic disorders are the most common causes of dizziness, at least in patients whose chief complaint is dizziness.[12] Ménière disease and acute labyrinthitis usually do not present problems in diagnosis; their abrupt onset, characteristic symptoms, and transient nature usually assure a speedy and accurate diagnosis. It should be noted, however, that although Ménière disease is perhaps the best known and most discussed of all the causes of dizziness, it is nevertheless a relatively rare disorder if appropriately stringent criteria are required for its diagnosis.

Benign paroxysmal positional vertigo is a self-limiting illness characterized by the occurrence of dizziness only in certain positions, usually only on lying down with one or the other ear dependent and on sitting up. The dizziness usually abates spontaneously after some seconds, and if the same position is assumed repeatedly over a few minutes, the dizziness progressively lessens and disappears. The most commonly identified cause for benign paroxysmal position vertigo is head injury, but in more than half the cases no specific cause can be found.[5] Usually the disorder is self-limiting, whether post-traumatic or idiopathic in origin. The diagnosis is made by physical examination if the Nylen-Bárány maneuver precipitates the symptoms and produces nystagmus. Following the appropriate movement, dizziness and nystagmus appear after a few seconds latency and disappear after a minute or two. The exact sequence, except that the rotatory nystagmus is to the opposite side, is repeated when the patient is returned abruptly to the sitting position. On repeated testing, the symptoms lessen and disappear after three to five trials.

Toxic neuritis occurs when medication adversely affects the vestibular system. The symptoms occur most often with analgesics and psychotropic medications, usually beginning within a few days of starting or increasing the dosage of the medication. Dizziness ceases after withdrawal or lowering the dosage.

Traumatic labyrinthine disorders are frequently encountered in psychiatric practice, especially as part of the postconcussion syndrome. Usually there is a history of head trauma with dizziness appearing within the first week or two thereafter. Often the dizziness is due to benign paroxysmal positional vertigo, but sometimes the pathophysiology is less clear.

Acoustic neuroma, a benign tumor of the eighth cranial nerve, rarely may cause dizziness by compression of the vestibular part of the nerve. Dizziness, which may be continuous, is seldom the initial symptom, and usually there are other abnormalities such as decreased hearing (especially for high frequency tones) on one side, palsies of nearby cranial nerves (V, VII, or X), and ataxia. Often the diagnosis is difficult and requires extensive testing with audiometry, electronystagmography, brain stem evoked response testing, skull x-rays, and posterior fossa contrast encephalography.

PSYCHIATRIC DISORDERS

Two types of dizziness commonly occur in patients with psychiatric disorders. The first is actually faintness, brought on most frequently in psychiatric patients by hyperventilation. Indeed, hyperventilation figures prominently as a cause of dizziness in all series of patients studied because of the complaint. Less frequently, faintness occurs in the setting of a sudden access of feelings, especially fear, anxiety, or anger. In these situations, the pathophysiology of the dizziness is well understood, as discussed in the first section of this chapter.

The other type of dizziness that is frequently encountered in psychiatric patients is best described as lightheadedness; for this sensation we have no acceptable pathophysiologic explanation. The description for this sort of dizziness is usually vague and sometimes bizarre, so that often the physician is left with no clear conception of the character of the symptom experienced by the patient. Psychiatric patients not infrequently report that the sensation is present continuously during the waking hours, a description that is unusual in most of the other varieties of dizziness for which some understanding of the pathophysiology exists. Very few organic diseases cause such continuous and prolonged dizziness. Lightheadedness is not specific for any particular psychiatric disorder but is seen often in conjunction with anxiety, depression, and somatization.

The Psychiatrist's Role in the Evaluation of Dizziness

The complaint of dizziness is so common in psychiatric patients that the psychiatrist must have some modus operandi for the evaluation of the complaint. First and most important is clarification of the symptom.

163

Careful questioning usually permits the physician to identify the symptom as one of faintness, vertigo, spatial disorientation, dysequilibrium, or lightheadedness. If after careful questioning the nature of the complaint remains uncertain, the psychiatrist may wish to use several of the maneuvers suggested by Drachman and Hart[2] in an effort to reproduce the symptoms. It is important, for example, that the psychiatrist identify the complaint as faintness, produced by a sudden drop in blood pressure on standing, and recognize that this may be the result of psychotropic medications. It is likewise important to know that the symptoms are due to hyperventilation—and it may be equally or more important as well for the patient to learn that overbreathing alone causes this frightening symptom. It is also essential for patient care that the physician ascertain that dizziness which began after head injury is not a conversion reaction or a "compensation neurosis" but can be reproduced along with nystagmus by the Nylen-Bárány maneuver.

Once the nature of the symptom is defined, the psychiatrist has several alternatives. It may be obvious that the symptoms are associated with medications, posture, specific movements, or hyperventilation, and the psychiatrist may conclude that more extensive evaluation is not required. On the other hand, it may be concluded that there is no ready medical or psychiatric explanation for the symptom presented and that extensive evaluation is warranted. In the latter instance, the psychiatrist usually refers the patient to another specialist for full evaluation, the choice of specialist being determined by the patient's specific complaint and by what is known of the patient's general state of health.

The psychiatrist is not expected to determine the etiology of dizziness in every, or even in most, instances. The psychiatrist is expected, however, to be competent in the evaluation of the symptom and to recognize those cases which need full neurologic, medical, or otologic investigation.

REFERENCES

1. Drachman, D.A.: Dizziness and vertigo, in Beeson, P.B., and McDermott, W. (eds.): Textbook of Medicine, ed. 14. W.B. Saunders, Philadelphia, 1975.
2. Drachman, D.A., and Hart, C.W.: An approach to the dizzy patient. Neurology 22:323, 1972.
3. Engel, G.L.: Fainting, ed. 2. Charles C Thomas, Springfield, Ill., 1962.
4. Fisher, C.M.: Vertigo in cerebrovascular disease. Arch. Otolaryngol. 85:529, 1967.
5. Harrison, M.S., and Ozsahinoglu, C.: Positional vertigo: Aetiology and clinical significance. Brain 95:369, 1972.

CHAPTER 11

DISORDERS OF MOTILITY

In this chapter we discuss in capsule form the disorders of motility most likely to be encountered by the practicing psychiatrist. Excluded from consideration are several entities that are unlikely to fall within the psychiatrist's scope; thus most of the peripheral neuropathies and neuromuscular diseases are omitted, as well as the severe hemiplegias and paraplegias. Movement disorders resulting from treatment with psychotropic medications are discussed in the following chapter.

PARKINSON DISEASE

The triad of bradykinesia (or akinesia), rigidity, and resting tremor is readily recognized as due to Parkinson disease. Diagnostic uncertainty arises occasionally, however, when the triad is not yet fully developed. Decreased motivation, diminished spontaneity, easy fatigability, constipation, and feelings of depression are often present and suggest a primary affective disorder, leading a few such patients to the psychiatrist. Careful observation and examination will reveal, however, clear signs of the disease—diminished blinking, mask-like face, soft monotonous voice, stooped posture, *marche à petits pas,* bradykinesia, difficulty initiating movements, rigidity, pill-rolling tremor—so that the diagnosis of Parkinson disease is seldom missed except through inattention.

Far more important to the psychiatrist are the psychiatric complications of recognized Parkinson disease. Depression, dementia, and untoward reactions to treatment are of greatest importance, but a much wider array of disturbances has been described.[11] Depression is common in patients with Parkinson disease, playing a clinically significant role in perhaps one third to one half of all patients. Controversy exists as to whether the depression should be considered an integral part of the disease picture itself or an epiphenomenon. Were it a psychologic reaction to the disease, one would expect the depression to lift with improvement in the motor disability, and this has sometimes been described. Marsh and Markham[33] found, however, that this is by no means a predictable occurrence, and depression persisted in many of their subjects despite improvement in other symptoms. Whichever position is correct, it seems clear that clinically significant depression occurs with greater frequence in Parkinson disease than in most other neurologic diseases. The frequency with which depression occurs in idiopathic Parkinson disease is of additional scientific interest because many of the psychotropic medications which produce parkinsonism as a side effect (see Chap. 12) result in depression as another unwanted toxic reaction.

The role of depression in the patient's symptomatology may occasionally be overlooked because of the prominence of the motor symptoms, so that patients must be questioned specifically about symptoms of depression. Recognition of depression in Parkinson disease is important because it often responds well to treatment with the tricyclic antidepressants. Marsh and Markham's study[33] suggested that the depression may not respond well to treatment with levodopa alone.

Although Parkinson's original description specifically emphasized the preservation of intellectual capacities in this disorder, recent studies have demonstrated the frequency of cognitive impairment.[26] Perhaps 40 percent of all patients experience some decline in cognitive capacities, most notably in tasks requiring comprehension and manipulation of novel stimuli. The severity of the dementia is correlated to a certain extent with both duration and severity of the disease. The dementia is the result of both subcortical and cortical neuropathologic changes. Tests of cognitive function often improve after treatment with levodopa is begun, but the improvement may not be a lasting one.[40]

In the past, psychiatric complications often resulted from the anticholinergic effects of the standard antiparkinsonism agents. With the decline in the popularity of these drugs in the treatment of parkinsonism, these reactions are rarely seen in patients with Parkinson disease per se; on the other hand, we often see anticholinergic toxicity in patients treated with both the antipsychotic agents and the anticholinergic antiparkinsonism agents.

Instead of central anticholinergic toxicity in patients with Parkinson disease, we now see many psychopathologic reactions to treatment with levodopa, the current medication of choice. Virtually any neuropsychiatric picture may emerge with treatment with levodopa—depression, manic states, acute delirium, dementia-like conditions, paranoid psychoses, severe agitation.[15] Such reactions occur both early and late in treatment, and they are more common in patients with some degree of dementia or with previous psychiatric dysfunction. They are usually related to the amount of levodopa prescribed, but the dosage producing toxicity varies widely from patient to patient. The neuropsychiatric complications of levodopa therapy can usually be controlled by lowering the daily dose. For many patients, however, this is undesirable and results in worsening of their parkinsonian symptoms. Miller and Nieburg[35] reported that l-tryptophan (2.5 gm/day) was effective in clearing the symptoms and signs of psychiatric toxicity, permitting continued treatment with levodopa. Depression secondary to levodopa has been successfully treated with the tricyclic antidepressants.

TICS AND HABIT SPASMS[43]

Tics occur in a variety of recognized neurologic and psychiatric disorders, in most of which they represent a minor rather than a major manifestation of nervous system dysfunction. They also may result from use of a number of drugs. In this section, however, we deal with these abnormal movements only as they constitute a specific and usually isolated complaint in patients who generally are regarded otherwise as healthy.

The terms tic or habit spasm are used interchangeably for movements in which the impulse toward movement is involuntary. The movements are usually brisk and sudden, irregularly repetitive, stereotyped, involve normally synergistic muscles unilaterally or more often bilaterally, and imitate purposeful, coordinated actions. They usually begin in the muscle groups about the eyes and mouth, and they may spread. To the observer, they may appear as blinks, grimaces, taps, coughs, or in many other forms. As with a wide variety of other abnormal movements, they disappear during sleep and may be strikingly influenced by emotional factors, being markedly increased under stress and reduced when calm and relaxed. These abnormal movements are to some degree under voluntary control, i.e., the subject can usually inhibit the movement for a while during which time the urge to repeat the movement increases strikingly. The person eventually gives in to the urge to perform the characteristic movement, and a variable period of relief follows during which the urge somewhat abates.

These movements most often begin in childhood and seldom appear for the first time in middle and late life. In many patients they come, last for a while, and then disappear. These of course do not usually come to medical attention. In others, the symptom is chronic, although there may be marked variability from month to month and year to year. Occasionally a young patient begins with what appears to be habit spasms but with time the disorder progresses until the typical signs of Gilles de la Tourette syndrome (vide infra) are seen.

Tics and habit spasms have never been classified comfortably as either neurologic or psychiatric in origin. Because there are no other abnormalities on neurologic examination and no neuropathologic lesion

167

has been identified, neurologists tend to regard the movements as functional. The degree of voluntary control that the patient retains over the movements fits with this as does their resemblence to other acts seen in compulsive disorders. On the other hand, no specific psychopathologic dysfunction has been identified in these patients, and indeed they often appear normal on psychiatric evaluation; nor has psychiatric treatment with a variety of modalities led predictably to improvement. The truth of the matter is that since neither specialty has a ready remedy to correct the disorder, each would like to see tics and habit spasms placed within the other's purview. Of interest to psychiatrists is the statement of Ferenczi (quoted by Weingarten[13]) that Freud said he believed an organic factor would probably prove to be responsible for tics.

Treatment is at best unpredictable. Environmental manipulation to reduce stress, supportive and uncovering psychotherapy, and minor tranquilizers in small doses may help but are seldom curative. Various behavioral therapy techniques have been used,[3,45] also with variable results.

SPASMODIC TORTICOLLIS[34]

This disorder may perhaps best be conceptualized as a habit spasm involving the muscles of the neck, producing rotation of the head, and often tilting the head to one side. The sternocleidomastoid and trapezius muscles are usually most prominently involved, but the deep neck musculature often participates, and contraction sometimes spreads to the face and to other truncal muscles. In certain respects, the movements may differ from habit spasms as described in the preceding section. Although most commonly clonic and arrhythymically repetitive, they are sometimes tonic and may resemble the movements of tortion spasms (vide infra). Some authorities regard them as a variety of tortion spasm. Also, they are not inhibited voluntarily as easily as other habit spasms, but the patient is often able to inhibit them with gentle pressure by hand or finger exerted in the direction opposite to the repetitive movement.

Most of what was said about the etiology of tics is true of spasmodic torticollis. Although it may occur secondary to recognized neurologic disease, in most instances there are no abnormalities either on neurologic or pathologic examination. On the other hand, psychologic explanations are equally unconvincing. In the series reported by Matthews and colleagues,[34] psychologic assessment revealed no deviation from normal concerning abnormal movements exerting a profound deleterious psychologic effect on the affected patients.

Matthews and coworkers[34] reported the prognosis in spasmodic torticollis to be unexpectedly poor. Only 1 of their 30 patients made a full and sustained recovery, although a few of the others experienced some improvement or gave histories of remissions and exacerbations. The usual modes of psychotherapy are generally ineffective as are psychotropic medications. Neurosurgical techniques usually fail to achieve complete relief; they also may result in considerable loss of function. Recently, biofeedback techniques have been tried,[12,24] and Korein and Brudny[24] stated that the possibility for significant improvement is greater than 40 percent when electromyographic feedback techniques are used. Unfortunately, the period of follow-up has been limited in most of these studies, as is inevitably the case for a new treatment modality. Longer-term studies are required before the place of biofeedback techniques in treatment can be assigned with finality. A favorable response to biofeedback would not, of course, resolve the question of etiology.

HEMIFACIAL SPASM (CLONIC FACIAL SPASM)[10]

This abnormality of movement, which occurs largely in middle-aged and elderly women, is limited to the muscles supplied by the seventh cranial (facial) nerve. It is usually unilateral, begins insidiously in the muscles about the eye, gradually spreads to involve all muscles supplied by the facial nerve, and increases slowly in severity. At first, the movements tend to be clonic, i.e., simple twitches, but with progression they may become so rapidly repetitive that they are virtually tetanic. Characteristically, they appear in episodes lasting from seconds to many minutes during which repetitive spasms occur. In severe cases, the spasms become almost continuous. Facial hemispasm may be accompanied by facial muscle weakness and may appear as a sequela to Bell palsy.

The movements differ in several respects from habit spasms. They are not under voluntary control and cannot be purposefully inhibited. They may, however, be precipitated by voluntary contraction of the facial muscles. Patients sense no feeling of compulsion to carry out the movements, and indeed often it is impossible to mimic the movements at will. Furthermore, the spasms may continue during sleep or even wake the patient from sleep.

Hemifacial spasm is considered by all to be a neurologic disorder, and there is nothing to suggest that it is functional in origin. The psychiatrist should be able to recognize the disease, however, because patients with a wide variety of movement disorders are referred for psychiatric assessment in the mistaken belief that they are psychologically induced. The exact site and nature of the neurologic lesion causing facial hemispasm is uncertain, and there may be several disorders which result in the same clinical manifestations. It is believed to be due to a lesion of the facial nerve itself, but the nature of the lesion is uncertain.

169

Rarely it results from a cholesteatoma or a neurofibroma directly impinging upon the nerve. Recently it has been suggested that hemifacial spasm is caused by normal or pathologic blood vessels that cross and compress the facial nerve at its point of exit from the brain stem.[31]

The disorder is chronic and slowly progressive, and it sometimes terminates with facial paralysis. No treatment has been proved effective, although of course any manipulation of the facial nerve which produces paresis will lessen the spasm, thus exchanging paresis or paralysis for spasm. When the syndrome is due to nerve compression, neurosurgical decompression may be therapeutic.[31]

TORSION SPASM (TORSION DYSTONIA, DYSTONIA MUSCULORUM DEFORMANS)[32,46]

This disorder is in many ways typical of those neurologic disorders, sometimes presenting with bizarre symptomatology, that have been differentiated from hysteria. Dystonia may be a symptom of many neurologic diseases (cerebral palsy, infantile hemiplegia, kernicterus), and in these instances it causes little diagnostic difficulty. It is another matter, though, when dystonia appears as an isolated symptom in an otherwise healthy person, as is usually the case.

The manifestations of torsion dystonia arise characteristically from prolonged but shifting muscle spasms that result in postural abnormalities and slow, twisting, involuntary movements. The truncal and proximal limb muscles are most often involved, but any muscle may participate. Initial symptoms, which are often a postural change in the trunk or one extremity or clumsiness in certain specific acts, may be intermittent, with the symptoms at first confined to certain anatomic regions. They may remain so limited, but spread to other areas is common, and in some patients virtually all the trunk and proximal limb muscles eventually are involved. When not too severe, rest or sleep may abolish the postures and movements (as may intravenous barbiturates), but with time postural fixations supervene which are not abolished even by sleep. The symptoms and signs are usually progressive, at least in the early years, but long periods of stability and even regression have been observed. The spasms can in no way be controlled voluntarily.

Torsion spasm is a rare disorder whose onset is most frequent during the years of childhood, although onset has been reported as late as the sixth decade. The family history is positive for dystonia in many patients, but negative in perhaps two thirds or three quarters. Many *formes frustes* of the disease have been reported in family members. The disease tends to be more severe and involvement more diffuse when the onset is in childhood.

The diagnosis is made on the basis of: (1) unusual sustained postures of the trunk and extremities; (2) involvement of these regions in slow, writhing movements due to shifting patterns of muscle spasms; and (3) positive family history.

No specific (or even nonspecific) neuropathologic lesion has been identified, nor has any specific neurochemical defect been found. Torsion spasm is thus one of the interesting group of diseases universally recognized as neurologic but in which the nature of the defect is totally unknown.

Early diagnosis is difficult, and mistaken diagnoses are many. Forty-three percent of the cases reported by Marsden and Harrison[32] had been diagnosed originally as hysteric; almost exactly this same figure was found as well in the series reported by Lesser and Fahn.[25] Torsion spasm is mistaken for hysteria because of the nature of the complaints and the uncertainty of the neurologic changes. Initial symptoms are often bizarre—impairment of walking forward but not backward, impairment of walking but not running, turning in of one foot only when walking, rotation of one hand only with writing. In addition, initial symptoms may be limited and be consistent with a presumed psychogenic disorder such as writer's cramp. Neurologic changes may be absent or unimpressive. Symptoms are often absent at the time of examination, or, on the other hand, the postural changes may be so unusual that it is at once thought to suggest a conversion reaction. Psychiatrists should thus learn to recognize the disorder so that they do not fall into diagnostic error.

Treatment is entirely symptomatic, and none has been predictably effective. Marsden and Harrison[32] suggested that psychotropic agents which induce parkinsonism are most effective in controlling the involuntary movements of torsion spasm. Electromyographic feedback techniques are helpful in some patients.[4] In a few, the dysfunction is so severe that stereotactic brain surgery is employed. Psychotherapy has been ineffective in alleviating the involuntary movements, but supportive psychotherapy may help the patient and the patient's family to adjust to the disease.[18]

CHOREAS

Choreiform movements are quick, phasic contractions of groups of muscles producing displacement of the body part. Most frequently involved are the muscles of the face, tongue, and extremities (especially distally), but muscles of the trunk or even the diaphragm may be affected. The involuntary movements are arrhythmic, asymmetric, and unpredictable; they are usually increased in situations of stress and diminished in quiet and repose; they disappear with sleep. Groups of muscles that are normally synergistic may be involved, and if so the affected person may

171

be able to conceal the abnormality to a degree by merging the choreiform movement into some common movement of postural adjustment or grooming. The patient is powerless to inhibit them.

Chorea, observed in many acute and chronic neurologic disorders, usually is easily recognized as but one manifestation of the primary neurologic disease. Choreiform movements are, however, a primary manifestation of two neurologic diseases which often come to the psychiatrist's attention.

Acute Chorea (Sydenham Chorea)

In this disorder, largely affecting children and adolescents, chorea is a manifestation of active or preceding acute rheumatic fever. The choreiform movements appear insidiously and progress over a few days, in some cases becoming severe and almost continuous. They may be predominantly unilateral. They are often accompanied by mental symptoms such as irritability, agitation, anxiety, fear, confusion, insomnia, and even hallucinations. In younger patients the disorder is easily recognized clinically, and the diagnosis is usually confirmed by laboratory evidence of rheumatic involvement. The disorder is usually self-limiting, but psychologic sequelae may persist in a few patients for many years.[19]

Sydenham chorea occasionally recurs in adult life or even appears then for the first time, almost always in women who are pregnant (chorea gravidarum).[26] Oral contraceptives have also been reported to cause Sydenham chorea, usually in patients who experienced chorea earlier in life.[44] It usually appears acutely sometime during the first half of pregnancy, and the choreiform movements may be accompanied by striking mental symptoms, especially fear, anxiety, panic, personality changes, irritability, depression, dysarthria, emotional lability, and hallucinations. In such instances, the bizarre movements may be mistaken for signs of catatonic schizophrenia, or the hyperkinesis for evidence of mania, or the whole episode for hysteria.[44] The mistaken diagnosis thus leads to inappropriate treatment. Careful analysis of the movement disorder should prevent such errors in every instance.

Treatment with barbiturates or minor tranquilizers is frequently successful in controlling both the acute chorea and the mental symptoms. There are no good long-term follow-ups on the psychiatric status of patients who have experienced chorea in adult life. Studies of patients who had Sydenham chorea in childhood and who have been evaluated many years afterwards disclose, in comparison to controls: (1) a high incidence of psychologic stress *prior* to the episode of chorea; (2) poor educational and vocational achievement subsequent to the chorea; and (3) a high incidence of neurotic and personality disorders many years later.[19]

172

Huntington Disease[7]

This is generally described as a hereditary disorder characterized by both dementia and choreiform movements. Symptoms usually appear in adult life but sometimes are seen earlier. The dementia is usually explained on the basis of both cortical and subcortical pathology; the chorea, on the basis of marked degeneration of the caudate nucleus and putamen. When both chorea and dementia are present from the onset, the diagnosis presents few problems. In addition, Huntington disease is inherited as an autosomal dominant with high penetrance, and thus the disorder almost always has been present in one of the patient's parents. Proof of this is at times difficult to obtain, however, for these families often deny or manage to conceal evidence of the disease in previous generations, and parentage is not always certain.

The psychiatrist is likely to come up against problems in dealing with these patients when the dementia precedes the chorea or when a nonorganic psychosis precedes or complicates the other manifestations of the disease.

Dementia occurs in virtually every case of Huntington chorea. In some it may precede the appearance of chorea by some years (and rarely the chorea may never appear). When the family history is known, the diagnosis is clear. When the family history is obfuscated, however, the physician must find other clues to reach the correct diagnosis. Caine and associates[9] studied the neuropsychologic features of the disease early in its course. They emphasized in their patients awareness of failing mental powers (in contrast to what is observed in most dementias); impaired ability to organize, plan, and sequentially arrange information; loss of finely detailed memories; marked difficulty recalling material on command, and impaired ability to initiate activities spontaneously. They suggested that these deficits were due to a loss of cortical function similar to that found with frontal lobe damage. Butters and associates[8] compared the cognitive changes in patients with recently diagnosed Huntington disease and with far advanced disease. In the recently diagnosed patients, they noted defects especially in the memory quotient, short term memory, and ability to search and retrieve from long term memory stores. With far advanced disease, more global defects were the rule. They suggested that memory deficits are early focal signs that precede more widespread intellectual deterioration. McHugh and Folstein[30] studied a group of patients with more advanced disease and suggested that three features of the dementia might alert the examiner specifically to the possibility of Huntington disease, even in the absence of chorea or a positive family history. These features are: (1) the early presence of a prominent psychic apathy and inertia that may worsen to an akinetic mute state; (2) "a slowly progressive dilapidation of all cognitive powers"; and (3) the absence of features specific for aphasia, alexia, apraxia, agnosia, cortical blindness, or Korsakoff-type amnesia. Unfortunately it is clear that neither of these studies pointed to neuropsychologic changes sufficiently specific to permit in and of themselves a diagnosis of Huntington disease.

In addition to dementia, patients with Huntington disease often experience psychotic episodes which cannot be attributed to their cognitive dysfunction. These episodes, often acute in onset, may appear long before the cognitive impairment, as well as when the disease is already well established. These psychoses take two forms: (1) a mood disorder, most frequently depression but rarely mania, that cannot be distinguished by its clinical features from manic-depressive disease and (2) a delusional-hallucinatory state with features resembling acute schizophrenia.[30] Both types may come on abruptly, persist for several months, and resolve spontaneously. The affective psychosis is reported to respond both to antidepressant medications and to electroconvulsive therapy (ECT). The delusional-hallucinatory state does not respond to treatment so predictably. In some, major tranquilizers appear to be effective and in others, antidepressants or ECT. Caine and coworkers[9] emphasized, on the one hand, the sensitivity of many Huntington disease patients to even small amounts of psychotropic medications, and, on the other, the need in others for large quantities of these medications for control of the psychotic symptoms. The major point about these psychotic episodes is that their usual course of remissions and exacerbations is distinctly different from that of the primary Huntington disease process (which is slowly progressive to death) and that they often respond well to psychiatric treatment.

GILLES DE LA TOURETTE SYNDROME

Shapiro and Shapiro[36] defined this syndrome as "a chronic, multiple-tic condition that begins in childhood and is characterized by involuntary, sudden, rapid, and purposeless movements and vocalizations that can include sounds, words, and coprolalia." Nowadays, it is considered by most to be the result of organic nervous system disease, this conclusion having been reached largely because (1) electroencephalographic abnormalities are frequent in the disorder, (2) psychologic testing often reveals patterns which are typical of organicity, and (3) recent studies emphasize the importance of genetic factors in the development of the syndrome.[20] Yet, the abnormal movements have many of the characteristics of compulsions.

The disorder usually begins in childhood with simple, involuntary, tic-like movements (vide supra). Involuntary utterances (resembling grunts, barks, or coughs) may also be present at the onset. With time, the symptoms spread to involve more and different muscle groups, and old stereotyped abnormal movements often drop out as new ones appear. The involuntary movements may assume greater complexity, coming to involve squatting, hitting, jumping, or touching. Athetoid and dystonic type movements sometimes appear. Involuntary utterances occur in virtually all patients, but coprolalia (often assumed to be the hallmark of the disorder) occurs in only about one half; echolalia also is not uncommon. The clinical picture is marked by changeability, not only in clinical signs but in severity. Although the disorder is chronic and usually progressive, it is not accompanied by mental deterioration.

When the syndrome is full-blown, diagnosis usually presents few problems. Early in its course, especially if symptoms are circumscribed, or later during periods marked by clinical variability, diagnosis may be difficult.[6] Diagnostic uncertainty is usually resolved, however, by repeated evaluations over a period of time.

The clinical manifestations are to some extent under voluntary control. Patients may with effort inhibit certain symptoms, but this is often balanced by an increase in other symptoms during this period of effort. The span of voluntary inhibition may be followed by an almost explosive outburst of the inhibited symptoms. In the past these characteristics have led some physicians to consider the abnormal movements of Gilles de la Tourette syndrome a type of compulsive neurosis. However, there is no evidence for specific psychologic conflicts in this disorder, and psychoanalytically oriented psychotherapy and behavior modification techniques have generally been ineffective in changing the course of the disease.

The waxing and waning of the symptoms and signs of Gilles de la Tourette syndrome have made treatment evaluation difficult. Haloperidol is the only therapeutic agent that has produced predictable improvement in any significant percentage of patients.[37] Even so, some patients do not respond favorably, and even in the responsive patient, control of the abnormal movements with haloperidol is often difficult to achieve, for side effects of the medication are common and sometimes limiting. Much effort may be required to achieve the best symptomatic control at a dosage level that does not produce unacceptable side effects.

PAROXYSMAL KINESEGENIC CHOREOATHETOSIS[23]

This disorder, which is both rare and odd, is manifested by brief, repetitive, stereotyped episodes of choreiform, athetoid, or dystonic movement and posturing that may be unilateral or bilateral. These episodes of involuntary movement are usually precipitated by movement, sometimes by a startle reaction; they generally last only a few seconds but may occur many times daily. These gyrations commonly begin in childhood or adolescence, sometimes even in infancy; some cases are familial.

The neurologic examination is characteristically unremarkable as is the electroencephalogram. Pathologic examination revealed no significant abnormalities in the one case studied. The episodes are usually well controlled by phenytoin (Dilantin), leading to the suggestion that this is a form of "reflex epilepsy," even though there are no EEG changes.

The paroxysms appear very bizarre, leading to their misdiagnosis as hysterical and to referral of these patients to psychiatrists.[42] Since the symptoms are abolished by phenytoin, it is important that psychiatrists recognize the disorder and institute appropriate treatment. Of the 10 patients reported by Kertesz,[22] one committed suicide and another experienced a depressive illness. Whether the depressions seen in paroxysmal kinesegenic choreoathetosis occur as a reaction to the disorder or whether they suggest an association between depressive illness and the disorder has not been explored.

ESSENTIAL TREMOR (FAMILIAL TREMOR, SENILE TREMOR)[13,14]

Essential tremor is a coarse or fine, rhythmic or arrhythmic tremor with a rate of 4 to 14 Hz. It is usually most striking in the upper extremities, especially in the hands, and involves the head less prominently; voice, jaw, and legs also may be affected. Typically the tremor is minimal or absent at rest and is brought out by movement. The shaking is usually most severe with certain specific actions, i.e., drinking (especially from a teacup), eating, and writing. Most patients report that the tremor worsens significantly whenever their movements are observed by others, such as when drinking from a cup or signing a legal document in public. Emotional stress of any sort accentuates the shaking.

The tremor may begin in childhood, old age, or anytime between. There is often a positive family history, and in such instances the pattern of inheritance is most consistent with an autosomal dominant mode. Hereditary factors are most consistently observed in patients with youthful onset. In most patients, the disorder is slowly progressive. For some, impairment in function becomes severe, but for most the tremor is more a troublesome annoyance and embarrassment than anything else. The neurologic examination is unremarkable except for the tremor. No specific neuropathologic lesion or neurochemical defect has been identified.

The tremor is *noticeable,* and therein lies the problem for many patients whose tremor is not otherwise significantly limiting. Often told by one and all that they are nervous, "up-tight," and have emotional problems, they often come to accept this valuation of themselves as accurate. In others, the tremor may be so severe that patients come to refrain from drinking, eating, or even signing their names in public;

embarrassment leads some patients to reclusiveness. In others, the relief from alcohol leads to excessive alcohol intake and dependence.

Psychiatrists should learn to recognize essential tremor at once on the basis of the history and by observation of the tremor itself. Often explanation is all that is needed therapeutically or explanation plus pharmacologic agents. Not infrequently, however, the psychiatrist finds emotional problems requiring specific psychiatric treatment as well, the not unexpected outcome of what for some patients has been many years of misapprehension about the nature of the disorder.

To date, only two substances have been identified which reduce the severity of this tremor—alcohol and propranolol. For many years, alcohol has been recognized as effective in reducing the tremor in many patients with essential tremor. When used sparingly and for specific activities, it has proved a useful medicinal agent for many. On the other hand, the dangers of using alcohol to treat such a chronic ailment are apparent, and in some patients the effectiveness of the relief obtainable from alcohol has led to dependence and abuse. The beta-adrenergic blocking agent propranolol (Inderal) has recently been found to afford relief comparable to alcohol in some patients[39] (often only to those same patients who are also helped by alcohol). With careful attention to its possible toxic effects, propranolol may be slowly increased to doses of 320 mg per day in efforts to achieve relief. Unfortunately, a number of patients with essential tremor fail to obtain significant relief with either alcohol or propranolol. Supportive psychotherapy is often important in the treatment of these persons.

RESTLESS LEGS SYNDROME[17,21]

Approximately 5 percent of the population experiences the symptoms of this syndrome to some degree; in a much smaller percentage, the symptoms are sufficiently distressing that they bring the patient to the attention of physicians.

The affected person describes a sense of disquiet in the legs, most severe between the knees and the ankles. The sensation is often reported to be a crawling or creeping feeling, neither burning nor pins-and-needles in quality, which is intensely uncomfortable. Many persons observe an inability to find words that convey the sensation accurately. The discomfort occurs only with rest and is likely to be most severe shortly after going to bed. It is accompanied by an irresistable need to keep the legs moving, so that most individuals get up and walk until the discomfort passes. Severity varies from mild annoyance to distress so intense that it leads to severe insomnia. The syndrome may appear from youth to old age, and there is much waxing and waning of symptoms with time.

Diagnosis of the restless legs syndrome is based upon the typical history as outlined above in the presence of a normal neurologic examination. A satisfactory explanation for the syndrome is lacking. The restless legs syndrome has been associated with uremia, diabetes, and previous gastric surgery;[2] other investigators have observed a close relationship to depression and anxiety,[17] and Lutz,[28] has recently blamed the symptoms on caffeine toxicity. For the time being it appears judicious to regard this as a discrete clinical syndrome of unknown cause, more likely to be organic than functional in origin.

Often explanation and understanding afford sufficient relief to these patients who have often been plagued by fears of major psychiatric disease because of the strangeness and bizarreness of their symptoms. In more severe cases, treatment before bedtime with anxiolytic agents is helpful. Although the antipsychotics have been reported to be useful in control of symptoms, their long term use should be avoided because of the danger of producing tardive dyskinesia in these patients whose symptoms persist over many years. Lutz[28] reported disappearance of the symptoms in several patients after abstinence from caffeine.

The syndrome of restless legs must be differentiated from akathisia (see Chap. 12). The following features of the syndrome usually permit a clear differentiation: (1) its occurrence in patients who are not taking antipsychotic agents (indeed antipsychotic agents have been reported to afford some measure of relief); (2) the appearance of the symptoms only with rest and their relief, often for significant periods, following activity; (3) the characteristic accentuation of symptoms after going to bed.

MYASTHENIA GRAVIS[38]

The common symptoms of myasthenia gravis—weakness, easy fatigability, blurred or double vision, difficulty swallowing and speaking, labored breathing with inspiratory difficulty—are the same as those encountered in many patients with primary psychiatric dysfunction. The prominence of these symptoms early in the course of myasthenia gravis, at a time when paresis is not apparent to observation, may result in the patient's being referred for psychiatric evaluation and treatment. The fluctuating course of the disorder, its tendency toward remissions and exacerbations, and the more frequent appearance of its generalized rather than bulbar forms in younger women, all add to the potential for diagnostic error by unwary physicians.

The salient clinical characteristics of myasthenia gravis are: (1) the increase in weakness in the involved muscles with repetitive contraction and (2) the restoration of strength partially or entirely with rest. Attention to these two features usually prompts the correct diagnosis. Not every patient with early myasthenia has attended to these aspects of symptomatology, however, and thus history alone does not always suffice. Testing of the weak muscles clinically usually confirms the presence of these features. The diagnosis is reached more easily on clinical grounds when the extraocular and other bulbar muscles are involved and thus the paresis can be observed directly. Other characteristics of the neurologic examination are the absence of pupillary changes and other signs of autonomic disease, the preservation of muscle stretch reflexes, and the preservation of normal sensory function.

The diagnosis of myasthenia gravis is confirmed by the demonstration of objective, measurable increase in muscle strength in response to anticholinesterase medications. Edrophonium chloride (Tensilon) 10 mg intravenously or 1.5 mg of neostigmine methylsulfate (Prostigmin) intramuscularly is the usual choice. The former has a rapid onset with peak effect in 3 to 5 minutes; the latter, a slower onset with peak in about a half hour. When there is a serious question as to whether the weakness results from myasthenia gravis or from functional causes, a double-blind procedure should be used, using both active medication and placebo. Since active drugs produce muscarinic side effects, however, even double-blind testing has drawbacks. In doubtful cases, electromyography with repetitive nerve stimulation, before and after anticholinesterase administration, is the procedure of choice to prove or disprove the diagnosis.

Myasthenia gravis is a disorder in which there is impaired conduction at the neuromuscular junction. Most authorities today relate myasthenia gravis to autoimmune dysfunction in which there is an antibody directed against the acetylreceptor on the muscle endplate.[16]

Treatment is dependent upon the use of anticholinesterase agents, adrenal corticosteroids, and thymectomy.[16,35] Most patients can now look forward to an active, useful life.

It is important that psychiatrists not mistake myasthenia gravis for functional psychiatric disease. It should be pointed out also that diagnostic errors go in the opposite direction as well, i.e., physicians sometimes mistake functional disease for myasthenia gravis and mistakenly treat the patients for myasthenia gravis for long periods. Since response to treatment is difficult to gauge, such errors are by no means incomprehensible.

Brolley and Hollender[5] highlighted the psychologic problems encountered in patients with proven myasthenia gravis. They pointed to problems in adjustment to long term illness, in treatment, and in dealing with fear and dependency. They observed as well the frequent exacerbations of weakness in these patients occasioned by emotional upsets. Depression also may be a significant feature in those patients who have been told by physician after physician that their complaints are functional in origin before the diagnosis of myasthenia gravis is reached.

PERIODIC PARALYSIS[1,29,41]

Although periodic paralysis is a well recognized clinical syndrome, a physician not familiar with the disorder might mistake any of its several varieties for hypochondriasis or a conversion reaction. For that reason, knowledge of the disorder is important for psychiatrists.

In contrast to myasthenia gravis, the episodic weakness in periodic paralysis usually comes on in the patient at rest (often when asleep), frequently when the rest has followed vigorous exercise and/or a meal high in carbohydrates. The weakness is gradual in onset, reaches its peak in 30 minutes or so, and lasts for hours or days if untreated. Limb muscles are more involved than those of the trunk, the proximal more than the distal. The bulbar muscles and the muscles of respiration seldom are involved seriously. There is often a positive family history. Neurologic examination during the episode usually demonstrates, in addition to weakness of the involved muscles, hypotonia, loss of muscle stretch reflexes, and preservation of sensory functions; at other times, the neurologic examination is entirely normal.

At least four varieties of periodic paralysis have been described which are associated with abnormalities of potassium metabolism: familial periodic paralysis, hyperthyroidism with periodic paralysis, adynamia episodica hereditaria, and congenital paramyotonia. In the first two disorders, the repetitive episodes of paresis are associated with hypokalemia; in the latter two, with hyperkalemia. In all these, the paralysis that occurs in response to small changes in serum potassium is often far more severe than that which is seen in normal subjects in response to shifts in the level of potassium. Myotonia is seen in both adynamia episodica hereditaria and congenital paramyotonia. In the latter, paralysis may be precipitated by cold. Another variety, normokalemic periodic paralysis, occurs with normal serum potassium levels, but it too is probably associated with some abnormality in potassium metabolism, because administration of potassium salts results in worsening. In addition to these disorders in which periodic paralysis is the chief manifestation, paralysis may be a manifestation of the hypokalemia that occurs in a variety of other medical disorders such as uremia, aldosteronism, and excessive use or abuse of diuretics.

Treatment of all the above described disorders depends on identifying and correcting the abnormality in potassium metabolism. Control of diet and potassium intake often effectively prevents recurrence of the episodic weakness. The psychiatrist will probably never be called on to manage therapy in a patient with periodic paralysis, but recognition of the disorder could sometimes be important.

REFERENCES

1. Adams, R.D., and Victor, M.: Myasthenia gravis and episodic forms of muscular weakness, *in* Adams, R.D., and Victor, M.: Principles of Neurology. McGraw-Hill Book Company, New York, 1977.
2. Baner, J.I., and Hurwitz, L.J.: Restless legs syndrome, with particular reference to its occurrence after gastric surgery. Br. Med. J. 4:774, 1970.
3. Barrett, B.H.: Reduction in rate of multiple tics by free operant conditioning methods. J. Nerv. Ment. Dis. 135:187, 1962.
4. Bird, B.L., and Cataldo, M.F.: Experimental analysis of EMG feedback in treating dystonia. Ann. Neurol. 3:310, 1978.
5. Brolley, M., and Hollender, M.H.: Psychological problems of patients with myasthenia gravis. J. Nerv. Ment. Dis. 122:178, 1955.
6. Bruun, R.D., and Shapiro, A.K.: Differential diagnosis of Gilles de la Tourette's syndrome. J. Nerv. Ment. Dis. 155:328, 1972.
7. Bruyn, G.W.: Huntington's chorea. Historical, clinical and laboratory synopsis, *in* Vinken, P.J., and Bruyn, G.W. (eds.): Handbook of Clinical Neurology, vol. 6. North-Holland Publishing Company, Amsterdam, 1968.
8. Butters, N., Sax, D., and Montgomery, K.: Comparisons of the neuropsychological deficits associated with early and advanced Huntington's disease. Arch. Neurol. 35:585, 1978.
9. Caine, E.D., Hunt, R.D., Weingartner, H., et al.: Huntington's dementia. Clinical and neuropsychological features. Arch. Gen. Psychiatry 35:377, 1978.
10. Cawthorne, T.: Clonic facial spasm. Arch. Otolaryngol. 81:504, 1965.
11. Celesia, G.C., and Wanamaker, W.M.: Psychiatric disturbances in Parkinson's disease. Dis. Nerv. Syst. 33:577, 1972.
12. Cleeland, C.S.: Behavioral techniques in the modification of spasmodic torticollis. Neurology 23:1241, 1973.
13. Critchley, E.: Clinical manifestations of essential tremor. J. Neurol. Neurosurg. Psychiatry 35:365, 1972.
14. Critchley, M.: Observations on essential (heredofamilial) tremor. Brain 72:113, 1949.
15. Damasio, A.R., and Caldas, A.C.: Neuropsychiatric aspects, *in* Stern, G. (ed.): The Clinical Uses of Levodopa. University Park Press, Baltimore, 1975.
16. Drackman, D.B.: Myasthenia gravis. New Engl. J. Med. 298: 136 and 186, 1978.
17. Ekbom, K.A.: Restless legs syndrome. Neurology 10:868, 1960.
18. Eldridge, R., Riklan, M., and Cooper, I.S.: The limited role of psychotherapy in torsion dystonia. JAMA 210:705, 1969.
19. Freeman, J.M., Aron, A.M., Collard, J.E., et al.: The emotional correlates of Sydenham's chorea. Pediatrics 35:42, 1965.
20. Golden, G.S.: Tics and Tourette's: A continuum of symptoms? Ann. Neurol. 4:145, 1978.
21. Gorman, C.A., Dyck, P.J., and Pearson, J.S.: Symptom of restless legs. Arch. Intern. Med. 115:155, 1965.
22. Grob, D. (ed.): Myasthenia Gravis. Ann. N.Y. Acad. Sc. 274:1, 1976.
23. Kertesz, A.: Paroxysmal kinesegenic choreoathetosis. Neurology 17:680, 1967.
24. Korein, J., and Brudny, J.: Intergrated EMG feedback in the management

of spasmodic torticollis and focal dystonia: A prospective study of 80 patients. Res. Publ. Assoc. Res. Nerv. Ment. Dis. 55:385, 1976.
25. Lesser, R.P., and Fahn, S.: Dystonia: A disorder often misdiagnosed as a conversion reaction. Am. J. Psychiatry 135:349, 1978.
26. Lewis, B.V., and Parsons, M.: Chorea gravidarum. Lancet 1:284, 1966.
27. Loranger, A.W., Goodell, H., McDowell, F.H., et al.: Intellectual impairment in Parkinson's syndrome. Brain 95:405, 1972.
28. Lutz, E.G.: Restless legs, anxiety and caffeinism. J. Clin. Psychiatry 39:693, 1978.
29. McArdle, B.: Metabolic and endocrine myopathies, in Walton, J.N. (ed.): Disorders of Voluntary Muscle, ed. 3. Churchill Livingstone, Edinburgh-London, 1974.
30. McHugh, P.R., and Folstein, M.F.: Psychiatric syndromes of Huntington's chorea: A clinical and phenomenologic study, in Benson, D.F., and Blumer, D. (eds.): Psychiatric Aspects of Neurological Disease. Grune and Stratton, New York, 1975.
31. Maroon, J.C.: Hemifacial spasm. A vascular cause. Arch. Neurol. 35:481, 1978.
32. Marsden, C.D., and Harrison, M.J.G.: Idiopathic torsion dystonia (dystonia musculorum deformans). A review of forty-two patients. Brain 97:793, 1974.
33. Marsh, G.G., and Markham, C.H.: Does levodopa alter depression and psychopathology in Parkinsonism patients? J. Neurol. Neurosurg. Psychiatry 36:925, 1973.
34. Matthews, W.G., Beasley, P., Parry-Jones, W., et al.: Spasmodic torticollis: A combined clinical study. J. Neurol. Neurosurg. Psychiatry 41:485, 1978.
35. Miller, E.M., and Nieburg, H.A.: L-tryptophan in the treatment of levodopa induced psychiatric disorders. Dis. Nerv. Syst. 35:20, 1974.
36. Shapiro, A.K., and Shapiro, E.: Subcategorizing Gilles de la Tourette's syndrome (letter to editor). Am. J. Psychiatry 134:819, 1977.
37. Shapiro, A.K., Shapiro, E., and Wayne, H.: Treatment of Tourette's syndrome with haloperidol, review of 34 cases. Arch. Gen. Psychiatry 28:92, 1973.
38. Simpson, J.A.: Myasthenia gravis and myasthenic syndromes, in Walton, J.N. (ed.): Disorders of Voluntary Muscle, ed. 3. Churchill Livingstone, Edinburgh-London, 1974.
39. Sweet, R.D., Blumberg, J., Lee, J.M., et al.: Propranolol treatment of essential tremor. Neurology 24:64, 1974.
40. Sweet, R.D., McDowell, F.H., Feigenson, J.S., et al.: Mental symptoms in Parkinson's disease during chronic treatment with levodopa. Neurology 26:305, 1976.
41. Talbott, J.H.: Periodic paralysis: A clinical syndrome. Medicine 20:85, 1941.
42. Waller, D.A.: Paroxysmal kinesegenic choreoathetosis or hysteria? Am. J. Psychiatry 134:1439, 1977.
43. Weingarten, K.: Tics, in Vinken, P.J., and Bruyn, G.W. (eds.): Diseases of the Basal Ganglia, Vol. 6. Handbook of Clinical Neurology. North-Holland Publishing Company, Amsterdam, 1968.
44. Weissberg, M.P., and Friedrich, E.V.: Sydenham's chorea: Case report of a diagnostic dilemma. Am. J. Psychiatry 135:607, 1978.
45. Yates, A.J.: Behavior Therapy. John Wiley & Sons, New York, 1970, pp. 192-206.

46. Zeman, W., and Dyken, P.: Dystonia musculorum deformans, *in* Vinken, P.J., and Bruyn, G.W. (eds.): Handbook of Clinical Neurology, vol. 6. North-Holland Publishing Company, Amsterdam, 1968.

CHAPTER 12

MOVEMENT DISORDERS ASSOCIATED WITH ANTIPSYCHOTIC AGENTS

The psychiatrist will doubtless see more movement disorders due to pharmacologic therapy than all the other types of movement disorders discussed in the last chapter combined. Abnormalities of movement arise occasionally from a wide variety of pharmacologic agents, psychotropic and otherwise, but the antipsychotic agents have a particular propensity for producing disturbances in motility. Indeed, Marsden and associates[11] in their fine review of this topic noted that the effect of antipsychotic medications on motor behavior is an important feature distinguishing them from sedative-hypnotics, antidepressants, and anxiolytic agents. The problem is of sufficient magnitude that the American College of Neuropsychopharmacology and the Food and Drug Administration some years ago joined forces to create a task force especially to investigate movement disorders due to drug toxicity.[1]

Four types of movement disorder are ascribed to the antipsychotic agents: (1) acute dyskinesia, (2) akathisia, (3) parkinsonism, and (4) tardive dyskinesia. All of the antipsychotic agents now approved by the United States appear to be capable of producing all four types of dyskinesia, although there are considerable differences among the individual agents in both the incidence and type of side effect that results.

ACUTE DYSKINESIA (ACUTE DYSTONIA)

The acute dyskinesias are the earliest of the extrapyramidal side effects to begin after institution of treatment with antipsychotic medications. They often appear only a few hours after administration of the drug; about half the cases of acute dystonia make their appearance within the first two days and almost all within a week after beginning therapy. They occur with greater frequency in the young than in the elderly, and more frequently with high potency than with low potency antipsychotic agents.

The dyskinesia consists largely of shifting, sustained muscle contractions, the clinical appearance varying with the distribution of muscles involved by the spasms. Involvement of the muscles of the eyes, face, oropharynx, jaw, and neck is most common. Oculogyric crises, adversive movements of the eyes, blepharospasm, grimacing, trismus, dystonic movements and protrusion of the tongue, torticollis, and backward arching of the neck and trunk are common. With wider muscle involvement, torsion movements of the trunk, writhing, and athetosis may be seen. Dysarthria, dysphagia, and even impairment of respirations sometimes occur. This movement disorder, usually appearing abruptly and without warning, may severely frighten the patient, as well as the patient's attendants. In addition, the intense, sustained muscle contractions may be very painful.

The acute dyskinesias can be aborted quickly by the slow intravenous administration of 0.5 to 2.0 mg benztropine (Cogentin) or 25 to 50 mg diphenhydramine (Benadryl).[14] Treatment with antipsychotics can usually then be continued by prescribing the antiparkinsonian anticholinergic drugs on a regular basis during the first 7 to 10 days of treatment, the period during which the danger of acute dystonic reactions is greatest. Because the overall incidence of acute dyskinesias is probably less than 5 percent, most authorities advise against the routine use of prophylactic antiparkinsonian drugs. Because of the high incidence of acute dystonic reactions in adolescents, however, and because many patients, once they have experienced an acute dystonic reaction, are loath to continue antipsychotics, Chiles[4] advised routine use of antiparkinsonian medications prophylactically in adolescents for the first 7 to 10 days of their treatment with antipsychotics.

Acute dyskinesia rarely may be confused diagnostically with tardive dyskinesia (vide infra). In these instances, the prompt response of the acute dyskinesias to intravenous diphenhydramine or benztropine and the lack of response of tardive dyskinesia usually clearly differentiates the two.[3]

AKATHISIA

Akathisia usually appears later in the course of treatment than acute dyskinesia, rarely within the first 48 hours after antipsychotics are begun. About half the cases of akathisia appear within the first month and nearly all within the first three months of treatment. Akathisia occurs in patients of all ages and is probably the most frequent of all the motor reactions to antipsychotic drugs. About 20 percent of patients on antipsychotics are said to develop akathisia at some time during the course of treatment, but the incidence has been placed nearer 50 percent when patients have been observed especially for its occurrence.[16] Its incidence is reported to be highest in association with the antipsychotic agents of high potency.

Akathisia refers not to any specific pattern of movement but rather to a state of motor restlessness which results from a subjective sense of inability to tolerate inactivity, a feeling of a constant need or desire to move. The sensations are reported to be markedly uncomfortable, although many patients have difficulty describing the nature of the discomfort with any precision. Patients with akathisia appear extremely restless, and in severe instances they keep themselves in constant motion—pacing, tapping, turning, changing postures. Severe insomnia may ensue. Akathisia is an infrequent manifestation of Parkinson disease itself, but when it is caused by antipsychotics, it is frequently associated with other manifestations of extrapyramidal dysfunction. Van Putten[16] found that 59 percent of patients with akathisia concomitantly experience akinesia, parkinsonian tremor, or dystonia. Thus, in the affected patient, one frequently observes the surprising association of extreme restlessness and bradykinesis.

From a diagnostic standpoint, there is danger of mistaking akathisia for psychologic dysfunction, because it is often difficult for patients to distinguish between the subjective states of restlessness and anxiety. This may be even more confusing, of course, in the severely disorganized psychotic patient who cannot communicate the nature of the sensation to others accurately. In these patients, akathisia may be interpreted as a worsening of the psychosis, leading to increasing doses of the antipsychotic drug which is itself the offender. The frequent association between akathisia and other extrapyramidal symptoms and signs often helps with its recognition. It may also be differentiated from anxiety or a worsening psychosis by its response to treatment. Increasing the dosage of antipsychotic agents leads to increasing symptoms and signs of akathisia, whereas withdrawal of antipsychotics results in its improvement and disappearance (although symptoms may abate slowly). Akathisia usually is reduced to some extent by the antiparkinsonian agents. Benztropine (Cogentin) or trihexyphenidyl (Artane, Pipanol, Tremin), in doses of 2 to 8 mg daily (given in one or two doses), is usually effective. Indeed the response to antiparkinsonian agents has been used as the criterion for the diagnosis of akathisia.[16]

PARKINSONISM

All of the symptoms and signs of Parkinson disease may result from treatment with any of the antipsychotic medications. Although parkinsonism is more likely to result from the use of some agents than from others, none appears to lack this potential entirely. Symptoms seldom have their onset during the first few days of treatment; but if symptoms of parkinsonism are going to occur, they appear within the first month of treatment in one half to three fourths of patients and in nearly all instances within three months. The overall incidence of parkinsonian symptoms is said to be about 10 to 15 percent in routine psychiatric practice.[11] It occurs in young and old, and individual predisposition is said to play a significant role. The incidence appears to be higher with the high potency antipsychotics.

The most common parkinsonian symptom to result from the antipsychotic agents is akinesia or bradykinesia. This is the earliest and often the only evidence of toxicity and consists of an overall diminution in movements (those which are both volitional and unconscious), hesitancy in initiating movements, and slowness in movements. Rifkin and coworkers[13] pointed out that it may be confused with the changes in motility that accompany depression, and if misdiagnosed as such, a significant therapeutic opportunity may be lost. In some patients, rigidity follows, further impairing the patient's motility. The characteristic "pill rolling" tremor of Parkinson disease comes on still later and is a relatively uncommon toxic effect of these medications.

The appearance of parkinsonian signs in patients taking antipsychotics seldom causes many diagnostic problems. In older patients, however, there may occasionally be a question as to whether the patient is developing true Parkinson disease or pseudo-Parkinson disease due to drug toxicity. In true Parkinson disease, tremor is usually a more prominent feature than is the case in most patients with drug induced parkinsonism. Asymmetry of symptoms and signs is likewise common in true Parkinson disease and uncommon in pseudoparkinsonism. If the antipsychotics are stopped, improvement in extrapyramidal signs usually follows in drug toxicity, and the symptoms and signs usually disappear within a few weeks. Occasionally signs persist for many months following discontinuance of the offending agents, but eventual total recovery is the rule.[9]

The symptoms and signs of parkinsonism due to drugs can usually be treated effectively with the anticholinergic antiparkinsonian agents, so that it is not necessary to discontinue the antipsychotics. Benztropine and trihexyphenidyl (in the dosages suggested for akathisia) or other antiparkinsonian medications are usually effective. Long term treatment is not usually required, and often the antiparkinsonian agents can be discontinued after several weeks without a recurrence of the toxic symptoms despite continuance of antipsychotics. This is an important therapeutic consideration, because it has been suggested that long term prophylactic treatment with antiparkinsonian medications may predispose patients to the development of tardive dyskinesia. It has also been suggested that tardive dyskinesia is more likely to develop in patients who develop parkinsonism in response to antipsychotic agents.[5]

188

TARDIVE DYSKINESIA

Of the extrapyramidal disorders caused by antipsychotics, only tardive dyskinesia need be feared seriously. The last of the extrapyramidal toxic syndromes to be recognized, it was believed originally to be a complication only of long term, high dosage treatment with the antipsychotics. Further observation has shown, however, that what is called tardive dyskinesia does not always appear only late in treatment, nor does it result only from high doses of medications. It can result from treatment with any of the antipsychotic agents now approved for use in the United States by the Food and Drug Administration.

The exact incidence of tardive dyskinesia is unknown. Simpson and Klein[15] made a "judicious" estimate that it appears in approximately 10 percent of patients on long term antipsychotic medications. Asnis and associates[2] reported, however, that signs of tardive dyskinesia can be detected in 43.4 percent of a population of outpatients maintained on antipsychotics. It seldom begins during the first six months of drug treatment, and Crane[5] stated that the greatest increase in incidence occurred between the second and fourth years of treatment. It appears reasonably well established that the incidence of tardive dyskinesia is greater in the old than in the young, and greater in females than in males. Crane[5] presented evidence that it is more likely to develop in patients who earlier had developed signs of parkinsonism in response to the antipsychotics. Others have suggested that it is more likely in patients with pre-existing organic brain disease, but the evidence for this is not yet convincing.

Tardive dyskinesia usually makes its appearance as a buccal-lingual-facial dyskinesia. So slight are the movements at first that its presence may be difficult to ascertain, but with progression a startling variety of movement abnormalities may be observed. In adults, dyskinesia is usually most severe in the orofacial region, with relative sparing of the musculature of the upper face. In children, tardive dyskinesia usually involves the muscles of the extremities, but diffuse involvement may be seen at any age. The movements may begin as restricted puckering, licking, sucking, chewing, or swallowing motions, but with the passage of time, almost any sort of involuntary movement may be seen, i.e., quick, darting protrusions of the tongue (the "fly-catcher" tongue); vermicular motions of the tongue; lip smacking; grimacing; choreiform movements of the facial muscles and those of the extremities resulting in torticollis; dystonic axial motions; chorea; athetosis; ballistic movements of the extremities; and tapping of the feet. Lordosis and pelvic thrust also may occur, with resulting postural and gait abnormalities. The involuntary motions are increased by anxiety, decreased by relaxation, and disappear during sleep. Attempts to inhibit the movements voluntarily in one area often appear to accentuate them elsewhere.

A similar but usually mild disorder in which the involuntary movements are limited to the orofacial area is seen not infrequently in elderly subjects who have never received antipsychotics. This has been attributed to old age, arteriosclerosis, senile dementia, and the edentulous state, but its etiology remains uncertain. A disorder which almost exactly mimics tardive dyskinesia also is seen sometimes as a complication of long term levodopa therapy for Parkinson disease.

The cause of tardive dyskinesia is not known, as is true for the cause of the other extrapyramidal complications of treatment with antipsychotics. It has been proposed, however, that the neuroleptics produce a chemical denervation of the dopamine receptors of the striatum, and that "after such prolonged chemical denervation some receptors may develop denervation hypersensitivity."[10] These hypersensitive receptors may then respond in an abnormal manner to even small amounts of dopamine that reach them and produce abnormal movements.

The course of tardive dyskinesia has not been determined exactly. It is known that discontinuance of the antipsychotic medication often leads to an immediate worsening of the movement disorder. Indeed, discontinuing the neuroleptic may bring the tardive dyskinesia to light, whereas none was apparent as long as the patient remained on medication. Although discontinuance of neuroleptics often leads to immediate exacerbation, if kept off the antipsychotic drugs some patients eventually improve. Marsden and associates[11] estimated that in patients who remain off the drugs, the movements will disappear with time in 20 percent, improve in 20 percent, and remain unchanged in the remainder. The prognosis for recovery is better in children and young adults.

In patients whose signs of tardive dyskinesia develop when antipsychotics are reduced or discontinued, reinstitution of treatment at previous dosage levels leads in most instances to disappearance or striking improvement in the abnormal movements. In patients whose tardive dyskinesia appears while receiving antipsychotics, increasing the dosage usually suppresses the involuntary motions for a time. This is, however, obviously a losing therapeutic gambit, for with the passage of time, ever increasing dosages of the antipsychotics will be required to control the dyskinesia.

Aside from suppressing the movements with the antipsychotics themselves, there is no treatment that will result predictably in disappearance or lessening of the involuntary movements of tardive dyskinesia. In this situation, Klawans[8] appropriately emphasized the importance of prevention. He listed six guidelines for minimizing the likelihood that tardive dyskinesia will occur. (1) Limit the subjects at risk, i.e., prescribe the antipsychotics only for psychotic patients in whom their use is clearly indicated and for whom other medications are ineffective; do not prescribe them for the control of neurotic anxiety or other symptoms which can be treated effectively with other medicaments. (2) Do not use anticholinergic agents in conjunction with antipsychotics except when they are clearly necessary and then only for limited periods of time, because this may increase the incidence of tardive dyskinesia. (3) Limit the dose of the antipsychotic drug, using only the minimal amount necessary to achieve the desired therapeutic results. (4) Limit the duration of treatment, i.e., always try to learn if a patient really requires long term or continuous treatment to maintain an improved clinical state. (5) Use drug free days whenever possible. (6) Follow patients closely and carefully so that the earliest signs of tardive dyskinesia may be detected. Quitkin and coworkers[12] emphasized especially the importance of this last point. They found that the first symptoms and signs of tardive dyskinesia rarely persisted when the movement disorder was detected early and antipsychotic agents were discontinued immediately. They concluded that the length of time symptoms have been present prior to discontinuation of drugs, not the age at onset or duration of treatment, may be the major variable that determines whether or not the syndrome is reversible. All of the preventive measures suggested by Klawans appear appropriate, but Crane[6] has highlighted the difficulty that exists in persuading psychiatrists to reduce the doses of neuroleptics and in getting them to discontinue neuroleptics when no longer needed or patently ineffective.

So long as large numbers of patients require long term treatment with antipsychotic medications, however, tardive dyskinesia will continue to occur and to require symptomatic treatment. Whenever tardive dyskinesia makes its appearance, obviously the most appropriate move, so far as the dyskinesia itself is concerned, is discontinuance of the offending medication. Unfortunately, this is not always best, when all factors are taken into consideration. The physician may conclude that the dangers of discontinuing the medication pose a greater threat to the patient's well-being than the tardive dyskinesia, and thus the patient is maintained on the antipsychotic medication and the tardive dyskinesia continues. In other patients, the antipsychotics are discontinued, and the tardive dyskinesia persists nevertheless. The physician must then seek other measures to relieve the involuntary movements.

An increase in dosage or reinstitution of treatment to suppress the abnormal motions temporarily is not acceptable symptomatic treatment unless the dyskinesia is severe and disabling. For most patients, the physician must turn to other pharmacologic agents in an attempt to provide relief. Klawans[8] suggested that drugs that decrease dopamine activity within the brain are likely to be most effective. He advised the use of reserpine (1 to 5 mg/day) and related drugs for relief of the abnormal movement. A variety of other substances (including ben-zodiazepines, deanol, lithium carbonate, and most recently choline[7]) has been reported to be beneficial in the symptomatic relief of tardive dyskinesia. The number of different agents suggested and the conflict-ing reports concerning their effectiveness all indicate that no currently available agent will predictably suppress the movements of tardive dyskinesia. The psychiatrist who is searching for an agent to provide relief from these movements would do well, however, to avoid the an-ticholinergic agents, all of which may result in worsening of the symptoms.

REFERENCES

1. American College of Neuropsychopharmacology-Food and Drug Adminis-tration Task Force: Neurologic syndromes associated with antipsychotic-drug use. New Engl. J. Med. 289:20, 1973.
2. Asnis, G.M., Leopold, M.A., Duvoisin, R.C., et al.: A survey of tardive dyskinesia in psychiatric outpatients. Am. J. Psychiatry 134:1367, 1977.
3. Beitman, B.D.: Diphenhydramine in the differential diagnosis of neuroleptic-induced oral-facial dyskinesia. Am. J. Psychiatry 134:695, 1977.
4. Chiles, J.A.: Extrapyramidal reactions in adolescents treated with high-potency antipsychotics. Am. J. Psychiatry 135:239, 1978.
5. Crane, G.E.: Pseudoparkinsonism and tardive dyskinesia. Arch. Neurol. 27:426, 1972.
6. Crane, G.E.: The prevention of tardive dyskinesia. Am. J. Psychiatry 134:756, 1977.
7. Growdon, J.H., Hirsch, J.J., Wurtman, R.J., et al.: Oral choline administra-tion to patients with tardive dyskinesia. New Engl. J. Med. 297:524, 1977.
8. Klawans, H.L.: Therapeutic approaches to neuroleptic-induced tardive dyskinesias. Res. Publ. Assoc. Res. Nerv. Ment. Dis. 55:447, 1976.
9. Klawans, H.L., Jr., Bergen, D., and Bruyn, G.W.: Prolonged drug-induced parkinsonism. Confin. Neurol. 35:368, 1973.
10. Klawans, H.L., and Weiner, W.J.: The pharmacology of choreatic move-ment disorders. Prog. Neurobiology 6:49, 1976.
11. Marsden, C.D., Tarsy, D., and Baldessarini, R.J.: Spontaneous and drug-induced movement disorders in psychotic patients, in Benson, D.F., and Blumer, D. (eds.): Psychiatric Aspects of Neurologic Disease. Grune and Stratton, New York, 1975.
12. Quitkin, F., Rifkin, A., Gochfeld, L., et al.: Tardive dyskinesia: Are first signs reversible? Am. J. Psychiatry 134:84, 1977.
13. Rifkin, A., Quitkin, F., and Klein, D.F.: Akinesia. A poorly recognized drug-induced extrapyramidal behavioral disorder. Arch. Gen. Psychiatry 32:672, 1975.
14. Shader, R.I., and Jackson, A.H.: Approaches to schizophrenia, in Shader, R.I. (ed.): Manual of Psychiatric Therapeutics. Little, Brown and Company, Boston, 1975.
15. Simpson, G.M., and Kline, N.S.: Tardive dyskinesia: manifestations, inci-dence, etiology, and treatment. Res. Publ. Assoc. Res. Nerv. Ment. Dis. 55:427, 1976.
16. Van Putten, T.: The many faces of akathisia. Comp. Psychiatry 16:43, 1975.

CHAPTER 13

HEAD TRAUMA

Head trauma, or more exactly brain trauma, is among the more common neurologic and neurosurgical emergencies. Most head injuries that occur in peacetime are of the closed or blunt variety and are due to traffic, sporting, or industrial accidents in which brain injury is the result of a sudden acceleration or deceleration of the cranial contents in relation to the cranium itself. Open head injuries, less common except in wartime, differ clinically in certain features from closed head injuries, but they need not be considered separately in this discussion of the psychiatric sequelae of cranial trauma.

Most closed head trauma of consequence results in sudden loss of consciousness. When unaccompanied by other neurologic deficits and followed by complete recovery, the condition is usually called cerebral concussion. When followed by neurologic abnormalities or residual intellectual deficit, it is usually called cerebral contusion or, in the presence of focal defects, cerebral laceration.

The unconsciousness that follows head injury may be brief or prolonged. In patients who survive and begin to recover (and this is the vast majority of brain injured patients), there may be a loss of memory for events just preceding the accident called retrograde amnesia (RA) and for events intervening between the accident and return of *persisting* awareness called post-traumatic amnesia (PTA). The patient may appear to be aware of and responsive to the environment for some time before the period of PTA is actually terminated. The duration of the period of RA tends to shrink or disappear as recovery proceeds. Miller[11] stated ". . . a claim of very prolonged retrograde amnesia (RA) demands careful examination," i.e., probably it results from functional and not organic factors. The extent of PTA may or may not lessen with recovery.

The duration of PTA has been found to be a good measure of the severity of brain injury sustained.[8,13] In patients whose periods of post-traumatic amnesia are 24 hours or less, complete return of intellectual capacities can be expected in many, perhaps in most.[9] In patients whose PTAs are greater than 24 hours, persistent intellectual deficits are far more common, and the patient who escapes without residual intellectual deficits is fortunate.

Several psychiatric syndromes have been reported to follow head trauma: dementia, psychosis, personality changes, neurosis, and the post-traumatic syndrome. As Lishman[9] pointed out, the occurrence of these syndromes depends not only upon the amount and location of brain tissue damage but also upon other factors—the patient's response to intellectual impairment, environmental factors, compensation and litigation, the emotional impact and emotional repercussions of injury, and the premorbid personality. All of these factors should be taken into account in evaluating the individual patient. Thus, both organic and psychologic factors are to be weighed in each patient with the psychiatric sequelae of brain injury.

PSYCHOSES

Both affective[8,11] and schizophreniform[8,9] psychoses have been reported to follow head trauma, sometimes immediately after the acute confusional state, sometimes after an interval of apparent improvement. The appearance of these psychotic illnesses in no way correlates with either the extent or the location of brain damage. In the patient's history or in that of the family, there are often hints that prior to the accident the patient had the proclivity to develop psychotic illness, but this does not rule out the possibility that trauma played some role either as cause or precipitant. Davison and Bagley,[3] in an exhaustive review of the literature relating brain disease to schizophrenia, concluded that trauma might play some causative role in the development of schizophrenia and not be merely a precipitant. However, with the affective psychoses, which are more frequent than schizophreniform psychoses following trauma, it appears more certain that the trauma usually has only precipitated a psychotic episode in a predisposed individual.

DEMENTIA

Although profound, enduring dementia can of course result from head injury, the surprising thing is its rarity,[9] especially in light of the frequency of severe head injuries in our society. Nevertheless, in patients with long PTAs (and in some with PTAs not so long), residual intellectual impairment is common, the cognitive defects correlating to a significant degree with both the extent and the location of brain damage. Cognitive impairment can usually be established with certainty on the basis of both mental status examination and psychologic testing. There is considerable evidence that, given equally severe trauma, younger patients tend to recover more completely than older ones. However, the extent of recovery remains to a significant extent unpredictable in the individual patient. Not infrequently severe impairment which has remained unchanged for several years after injury may be followed by significant recovery. This delayed improvement has been attributed among other things to the spontaneous lifting of an unrecognized, masked post-traumatic depression and to a change in motivation perhaps engendered by changed environmental circumstances, but a scientifically based generally acceptable explanation is lacking.

Progressive dementing disease has not been proved to occur as a result of head injury, except in boxers who are subject to repeated trauma. In boxers, dementia may become apparent and progress after the person's sports career, and thus head trauma, has ceased. Otherwise, if progressive dementia appears following head trauma, it should be presumed to have antedated the trauma but to have been unrecognized.

PERSONALITY CHANGES

Many changes in personality have been ascribed to head injury, but only two of these appear significantly related to either the extent or location of the brain damage: (1) the so-called frontal lobe syndrome[2,8-10] and (2) reduced control of hostility.[5,9]

Frontal Lobe Syndrome

The frontal lobe syndrome includes several features—a loosening of inhibitions (especially in sexual areas), lack of concern for others, inability to plan ahead, failure to predict the consequences of actions, and a lack of concern about the consequences of actions. These manifestations, often coupled with a euphoric "don't care" attitude and a denial of the presence or severity of the dysfunction, are difficult to measure. Their appearance is closely related to the extent of brain damage. Nevertheless, the syndrome may occur in the absence of cognitive impairment as measured by the conventionally used tests, and it may result from damage involving areas of the brain other than the frontal lobe. The syndrome is among the most difficult therapeutic and management problems confronting the psychiatrist, yet it has been largely neglected in contemporary psychiatric texts.

Blumer and Benson[2] recently published an excellent summary of the personality changes that follow significant frontal lobe damage. They emphasized two types of change, described as "toward apathy and indifference" and "toward puerility and euphoria." The first they termed "pseudodepressed"; the second, "pseudopsychopathic"; they also noted that admixtures of the two occur more frequently than pure types. Luria,[10] who also has studied the topic extensively, described two main symptoms: (1) a disturbance in the complex forms of active, purposeful behavior, including a loss of initiative and incentive that may extend to almost complete apathy; and (2) a disturbance in the patient's critical attitude toward the self, with a general disinhibition and an inability to predict or be concerned with the consequences of his or her behavior. Luria's two symptom complexes correspond closely to the pseudodepressed and pseudopsychopathic types described by Blumer and Benson.

The key to the clinical recognition of these disorders lies in the prefix "pseudo." The apathetic disinterested withdrawal of these patients often suggests a depressive illness, and the patient may even, for lack of a better word, complain of depression, but careful scrutiny reveals more an absence than an access of affect. As Hecaen and Albert[6] noted: "A disorder of activity, rather than of affectivity is the hallmark" of frontal lobe disease. Similarly, the pseudopsychopathic aspects are poor imitations of the real thing. Absent is the cunning manipulativeness of the psychopath; in its place are found only naive, crude attempts to gratify wishes immediately. For example, one of our recent patients, wishing to obtain a favored drug, stole a physician's prescription pad in order to provide himself with a forged prescription. Our patient, however, took the pad with him to the pharmacy, wrote the prescription within view of the pharmacists, and signed his own name to the prescription to which the physician's name was affixed, and was promptly taken into custody by the police.

Luria[10] separated the psychologic defects due to frontal lobe damage into the following categories: (1) disturbance in the regulation of activity, which includes limited attention span, easy distractibility, and an inability to mobilize energy or to program action; (2) disturbance in the regulation of movements, with particular difficulty learning and performing complex, new programs of movement; (3) disturbance of memory, especially evident in attempts to memorize new material and reproduce it selectively; (4) disturbance of intellect manifested particularly by a constriction of interests and concerns; (5) disturbance of emotional background—apathy, indifference, or euphoria.

As might be predicted from the character of the symptoms described, such dysfunction is difficult to measure. The most frequently used tests of cognitive function may reveal little if any that is abnormal. If frontal lobe damage is suspected, the testing psychologist must be informed so that more appropriate tests can be chosen. Often then the psychologist will be able to uncover evidence which specifically suggests frontal lobe damage through choice of specific subtests of the Halstead-Reitan bat-

196

tery, difficult tests of new learning and retention such as Kimura's recurring figures test and the analogous visual verbal memory test, the Wisconsin Card Sorting Test, some of Luria's tasks of motor alternation and sequencing, and tests of verbal fluency such as asking the patient to name within a limited period as many words as possible beginning with a given letter.

Episodic Aggressiveness and Violence

Sometimes recurrent episodes of aggressive and violent behavior occurring upon little or no provocation can be ascribed to brain trauma. The appearance of such behavior after head injury, in a person who did not behave in such a fashion before the trauma, certainly suggests a causal relationship. Nevertheless, this syndrome is a rare sequela of brain trauma and one less predictably related to the extent and severity of brain damage than is either dementia or the frontal lobe syndrome. It may occur in patients who lack other evidence of neurologic dysfunction on either neurologic or laboratory examination. It has been ascribed to focal damage to the temporal lobes or to the limbic-hypothalamic connections.

Although episodic violence (or episodic dyscontrol, as some have called it) is a rare phenomenon after head injury, trauma is found to play an important etiologic role in groups of patients who are studied specifically because of their episodic dyscontrol. In Elliott's series,[5] temporal lobe epilepsy (itself often caused by brain trauma) was the most frequently identified cause for episodic violence, with brain trauma (not associated with epilepsy) the second most frequently identified offender. There are, however, many patients with the episodic dyscontrol syndrome who have no evidence, historically or clinically, of neurologic dysfunction and whose symptoms therefore are attributed to psychogenic factors.

Personality changes that are less likely to be correlated with evidence of brain tissue injury include persistent fluctuating depression, anxiety, irritability, and obsessionality. These traits merge indistinguishably into the post-traumatic syndrome described below.

POST-TRAUMATIC NEUROSIS AND THE POST-TRAUMATIC SYNDROME[8,9,11,12]

These are often considered and discussed as separate entities, but because we are unable to distinguish between them on either clinical or other grounds with certainty, we will treat them as a single entity, most appropriately described as the post-traumatic syndrome. Major symptoms usually include headache, dizziness (usually too imprecise in its description to be called vertigo), irritability, emotional lability, sensitivity to noise, anxiety, complaints of poor memory, and impaired concentration. These symptoms occur in many patients just after the trauma; in some, the symptoms may be explained by slowed cerebral circulation or by benign paroxysmal positional vertigo (see Chap. 10), but in most patients there are no neurologic deficits and the acute symptoms are believed to result from nonspecific effects of the trauma. In most patients, the symptoms quickly recede and disappear. In some, however, such symptoms persist, worsen, or even are augmented by further complaints such as fatigue, anhedonia, impotence or frigidity, persistent depression, insomnia, nightmares, phobias, and obsessions. The clinical picture that emerges is one of a symptom complex fitting no recognized pattern except that of the post-traumatic syndrome. Certainly the symptom complex does not conform to any of the recognized syndromes of organic brain disease, nor does it conform to the usually accepted categories of psychiatric dysfunction.

The physician's first responsibility in such instances is, of course, to rule out a treatable organic disorder, but with these polymorphous symptoms this is an unlikely possibility. The neurologic examination is usually within normal limits as are the EEG, CT-scan, and other diagnostic procedures. Mental status evaluation most often reveals a reluctant, poorly cooperative subject who is anxious, irritable, complaining, demanding, and depressed. Energy level is low, and the patient appears to put forth little effort to answer questions fully and accurately. Formal tests to evaluate memory, mathematical ability, fund of information, and abstraction ability are often poorly performed, but the patient's ability to catalog symptoms, provide details of diagnostic procedures already performed and of treatment failures, and present an accurate account of physicians visited in correct temporal order fail to support an organic basis for the cognitive deficits demonstrated by the routine, stereotyped questions.

Psychologic testing may reveal evidence of "organic" dysfunction (as would be expected from the mental status examination), but the psychologist and psychiatrist should look at the evidence critically. In the post-traumatic syndrome, performance on psychologic testing is usually uneven and the impairment spotty, not conforming well to patterns seen in established organic syndromes. Incongruence in performance of tasks requiring similar brain capacities is often marked along with a lack of fit between interview and test performance. The evidence supplied by psychologic testing must be appraised by the psychiatrist just as all other observations must be.

There is still much controversy as to whether the post-traumatic syndrome is psychogenic in origin, due to brain damage, or the result of psychogenic and organic factors working concurrently. The bulk of evidence suggests that long-continued symptoms of the post-traumatic syndrome are not the result of brain tissue injury.

The symptoms of the post-traumatic syndrome do not correlate either with the severity of the trauma or with the extent of brain damage.[8,9,11,12] Indeed, the converse is true! The post-traumatic syndrome is rare in patients with serious brain damage and common in those in whom no brain damage can be demonstrated. Equally telling is the observation that virtually identical symptoms (save for the location of the pain) can be seen after trauma which does not involve the cranium at all. Twin studies have also shown a close concordance between symptoms in injured and noninjured twin pairs, further suggesting that neural injury is not the decisive factor in determining the symptoms.[4] Lastly, the prominence of this syndrome in persons who are litigants for financial compensation cannot be ignored. Miller[11] observed that the syndrome "is hardly ever seen after injuries sustained on the hunting field, while playing rugby football, or in the home. Yet the syndrome is encountered in a persistent form in more than half of all patients who sustain injuries entirely similar from the physical point of view at work or in traffic accidents." Miller may have been observing a society in which liability insurance was less pervasive than in the United States today. According to him, the most significant features in the persistence of the post-traumatic syndrome are that in the patient's view someone else is at fault and financial compensation is at least a possibility. Miller[12] has also argued compellingly that much of what is called the post-traumatic syndrome is actually simulation or malingering.

There is little evidence to support an organic neural etiology for the syndrome. Although relatively slight amounts of trauma can produce microscopic neuropathologic changes, the symptoms in this syndrome are entirely out of keeping with the amount of neuropathologic damage which might even generously be estimated. To say that the post-traumatic syndrome is probably not the result of organic brain damage is not, however, to say that it is clearly psychogenic in origin. There is no evidence that most patients with the post-traumatic syndrome were neurotic or were otherwise limited in their adaptive capacity before injury. Nor is there evidence that such patients are unconsciously (or even not so unconsciously) cultivating their symptoms until financial compensation is made. Some patients certainly do get better when a financial settlement is reached and litigation is ended, but many fail to improve and their suffering does not abate. Certainly, there is no evidence that psychiatric treatment is effective in these patients, even when secondary gain is not apparent and there seems to be cooperation. We admit, therefore, that although the evidence is against an organic etiology, the evidence in favor of a psychogenic etiology is far from compelling. The post-traumatic syndrome remains what Sir Aubrey

Lewis[7] called it in 1942—"that common, dubious, psychopathic condition—the bugbear of the clear-minded doctor and lawyer."

SUMMARY

In summary, head trauma is followed by a number of psychiatric sequelae. Some, particularly dementia and certain types of personality change, are clearly the result of brain damage. Others, most notably the post-traumatic syndrome, are unrelated so far as can be established to either the extent or severity of brain damage. In these, psychogenic rather than organic factors are usually implicated etiologically, but our knowledge of these syndromes remains incomplete. As Lewis[7] stated in the same paper: "Is it due to structural damage or is it psychogenic? The insistence upon this is understandable, but fallacious; understandable, because the somatic pathology of any disorder is of prime importance, and because so many social issues such as attributability and pension rights depend upon the answer to the question; fallacious because it ignores the real state of affairs at present, and asks us to say 'Yes' or 'No' to a question often unanswerable in that form."

REFERENCES

1. Bach-y-Rita, G., Lion, J.R., Climent, C.E., et al.: Episodic dyscontrol: A study of 130 violent patients. Am. J. Psychiatry 127:1473, 1971.
2. Blumer, D., and Benson, D.F.: Personality changes with frontal and temporal lobe lesions, in Benson, D.F., and Blumer, D. (eds.): Psychiatric Aspects of Neurological Disease. Grune and Stratton, New York, 1975.
3. Davison, K., and Bagley, C.R.: Schizophrenia-like psychoses associated with organic disorders of the central nervous system: A review of the literature. Brit. J. Psychiatry Special Publication No. 4:113, 1969.
4. Dencker, S.J.: Closed head injury in twins. Arch. Gen. Psychiatry 2:569, 1960.
5. Elliott, F.A.: The neurology of explosive rage. The dyscontrol syndrome. Practitioner 217:51, 1976.
6. Hecaen, H., and Albert, M.L.: Disorders of mental functioning related to frontal lobe pathology, in Benson, D.F., and Blumer, D. (eds.): Psychiatric Aspects of Neurological Disease. Grune and Stratton, New York, 1975.
7. Lewis, A.: Discussion on differential diagnosis and treatment of postcontusional states. Proc. Roy. Soc. Med. 35:607, 1942.
8. Lishman, W.A.: Brain damage in relation to psychiatric disability after head injury. Brit. J. Psychiatry 114:373, 1968.
9. Lishman, W.A.: The psychiatric sequelae of head injury: a review. Psychol. Med. 3:304, 1973.
10. Luria, A.R.: Frontal lobe syndromes, in Vinken, P.J., and Bruyn, G.W. (eds.): Handbook of Clinical Neurology, Vol. 2. North-Holland Publishing Company, Amsterdam, 1969.
11. Miller, H.: Mental sequelae of head injury. Proc. Roy. Soc. Med. 59:257, 1966.

12. Miller, H., and Cartlidge, N.: Simulation and malingering after injuries to the brain and spinal cord. Lancet 1:580, 1972.
13. Russell, W.R., and Smith, A.: Post-traumatic amnesia in closed head injury. Arch. Neurol. 5:4, 1961.

CHAPTER 14

OTHER NEUROLOGIC DISORDERS IMPORTANT FOR THE PSYCHIATRIST

ACUTE INTERMITTENT PORPHYRIA[43,46]

This long recognized disorder of porphyrin metabolism excites clinical interest far beyond that warranted by its frequency. The vagaries of its clinical manifestations result in its frequently being misdiagnosed,[4] so much so that acute intermittent porphyria has been called the little mimicker (in contrast to the great mimicker—syphilis). The varied features of the disease result in patients being seen by internists, surgeons, neurologists, neurosurgeons, and psychiatrists; each specialist must be attuned to the guises in which it appears.

Acute intermittent porphyria usually makes its clinical appearance between the second and fifth decades, more often in women than in men. Three aspects of its clinical presentation predominate: (1) abdominal pains; (2) polyneuropathy; (3) brain dysfunction. The abdominal pain is often severe, closely resembling that of an acute abdomen and leading to fruitless laparotomies. The recurrent nature of the pain, the absence of abnormal findings by laparotomy, and the association with other features of the disease eventually point to the correct diagnosis. The polyneuropathy involves predominately the motor pathways innervating the extremities, but the cranial nerves and those supplying the muscles of respiration can be affected. Profound weakness sometimes occurs with paralysis of respiration, swallowing, and extraocular movements.

Brain dysfunction can occur in virtually any form—delirium, headaches, generalized or focal seizures, aphasia, apraxia, visual abnormalities, or memory loss. Psychiatric manifestations have assumed almost every pattern—anxiety, excitement, depression, uncontrollable agitation, and schizophreniform psychoses (paranoid, catatonic). The psychiatric features are often inconsistent with a diagnosis of any of the well recognized psychiatric syndromes.

The disorder is episodic, frequently with abrupt onset and equally abrupt resolution. The patient may be asymptomatic and without signs of neurologic or psychiatric dysfunction during the periods of remission. Diagnosis is established by the demonstration of abnormal patterns of porphyrin excretion in the urine during exacerbations. There is no specific treatment, but chlorpromazine has been reported to alleviate some of the symptoms, and propranolol in large doses has recently been reported to be effective in the acute exacerbations.[6] Medical support is of prime importance and may be life saving in cases with respiratory paralysis.

Many patients with acute intermittent porphyria are referred for psychiatric evaluation not only because of the recognized psychiatric manifestations of the disease, but because the kaleidoscopically changing neurologic symptoms and signs often suggest a diagnosis of hysteria. The psychiatrist needs to recall that whenever an inexact or changing pattern of neuropsychiatric dysfunction emerges in a patient with recurrent bouts of abdominal pain or a primarily motor peripheral neuropathy, the diagnosis of acute intermittent porphyria should be considered. The psychiatrist should also be aware that exacerbations of acute intermittent porphyria are not only precipitated by such well recognized agents as barbiturates, sulfonamides, and griseofulvin but also by a number of other medications likely to be encountered by the psychiatrist in daily practice—chlordiazepoxide, meprobamate, phenytoin, glutethimide, imipramine and ergot preparations.

PAIN SYNDROMES

Meralgia Paresthetica[38,40]

Neuropathy involving the lateral femoral cutaneous nerve results in a specific pain syndrome usually called meralgia paresthetica. This nerve supplies the skin over the lateral aspect of the thigh and in its peripheral course is exposed to pressure and trauma which are thought to give rise to the neuropathy. The usual complaints are burning or aching pain, paresthesias, hyperesthesia, and numbness over the area of cutaneous distribution of the nerve, and a reduction in cutaneous sensation in the same area is found on neurologic examination.

Meralgia paresthetica occurs more often in men than in women, is more frequent in obese subjects, and is reported to be provoked by wearing gun belts, tight corsets or casts, and by pregnancy. The disorder is benign and usually no treatment is needed, but occasionally nerve infiltration with local anesthetic or even surgical division of the nerve may be required to relieve the pain. The limited and somewhat unusual distribution of the discomfort may lead to its being misdiagnosed as a functional disorder.

Tabes Dorsalis[35]

Most young psychiatrists probably have never seen a patient with tabes dorsalis. Even so, if they should encounter a tabetic patient with the full complement of classic neurologic symptoms and signs, there is not much likelihood that the diagnosis would be missed. Rarely, however, tabes may be manifested by lightning pains alone. Lightning pains are usually described in florid and sometimes inexact terms, so that they might be mistaken for a manifestation of hysteria by the physician who fails to recognize the distinctive characteristics of this variety of pain.

The lightning pains of tabes dorsalis usually occur in attacks. Although the individual episode of pain may last only for a few seconds, the pain may recur many times during an attack which may persist for hours or days. The pains are most intense in the lower extremities. Although they may move from place to place, they tend to be localized to one spot during a single attack. The discomfort does not radiate but is limited to a circumscribed area often no larger than a coin. The pain is described as being of high intensity and having a jabbing, piercing quality, as though coming from the outside straight into the painful area (as though the patient were struck there by lightning). The skin in the afflicted area often becomes hyperesthetic and sometimes even hyperemic.

Early in the course of tabes dorsalis both the blood and spinal fluid usually are strongly positive for syphilis. With the passage of a time, however, the spinal fluid reagin tests often revert to normal, and the fluorescent treponemal antibody absorption test or the Treponema pallidum immobilization test may be required to prove nervous system involvement. In addition there are usually striking neurologic abnormalities (Argyll Robertson pupils, areflexia, severely impaired appreciation of position and deep pain sensations). In rare instances, however, neurologic changes may be lacking, and the correct diagnosis then rests upon recognition of the distinctive characteristics of the pain.

Herpes Zoster

When herpes zoster follows its expected clinical course—radicular pain followed in a few days by vesicular eruptions within the involved dermatome—there is seldom any problem in correct diagnosis. When, however, the pain is unusually prolonged before the appearance of the rash, or when the pain is unusually severe or is described imprecisely, or when the rash is inconspicuous and goes unnoticed, diagnostic difficulties ensue.

Herpes zoster is due to infection of the posterior sensory root ganglion and the sensory nerve with the varicella virus. Usually a single root is involved unilaterally, most commonly in the thoracic region. The trigeminal ganglion and nerve, especially the ophthalmic branch, are the most frequently involved of the cranial nerves. The incidence of herpes zoster rises with age.

Symptoms usually begin with a high intensity pain, burning and lancinating in character, along the dermatome distribution of the involved nerve. A vesicular eruption, limited to the skin of the involved dermatome, generally follows within three or four days, but occasionally there is a longer delay. Neurologic examination may reveal impaired appreciation of all sensory modalities over the involved dermatome plus marked hypesthesia (so-called anesthesia dolorosa). Accompanying motor impairment is said to be rare but recently has received increasing attention in the neurologic literature. The disorder is usually self-limiting, and, except when the eye is involved, treatment is limited to analgesics and topical ointments for the skin lesions.

The acute disorder is sometimes followed by post-herpetic neuralgia, a sequela which is more common in the older than in the younger patient. With post-herpetic neuralgia, the patient experiences a constant burning, searing pain throughout the involved dermatome, frequently made even worse by sudden jolts of pain which may be set off by sensory stimulation of trigger areas on the skin. The severity of the pain and its chronicity may lead to serious depression and inanition. The danger of narcotic addiction is a serious threat in these patients, even though narcotics often fail to afford significant relief. Combined treatment with carbamazepine (Tegretol) and the tricyclic antidepressants has been reported to relieve the pain in a large proportion of patients.[16] Whether the reported response is due to the anticonvulsant and antidepressant properties of these medications or to some other pharmacologic effects is unknown. Pilowski[31] emphasized the importance of personality assessment in the planning of treatment programs for these patients.

SYSTEMIC LUPUS ERYTHEMATOSUS[9,15,18]

Systemic lupus erythematosus (SLE) is not, of course, primarily a disease of the nervous system. The frequency of its neuropsychiatric involvement is such, however, that it is appropriate to discuss its neuropsychiatric complications in this volume. The brain and the peripheral nerves may be involved directly by the pathologic changes typical of lupus erythematosus; hypertension and uremia, both of which may secondarily impair brain function, are frequent manifestations of the disorder; and, finally, most patients with SLE are treated with corticosteroids, which sometimes produce a toxic psychosis or an electrolyte imbalance sufficient to impair brain function. The possible varieties and combinations of nervous system dysfunction in SLE are thus virtually limitless.

The exact frequency of neural involvement in lupus is uncertain, so different are the patient groups and methods employed in the various studies. It is probably safe to say that a minimum of 50 percent of all patients with lupus erythematosus experience neuropsychiatric complications sometime in the course of their disease and that of these, about half develop signs of organic impairment of the highest integrative functions.[9] Less common neurologic manifestations include seizures, cranial nerve dysfunctions, long-tract signs including hemiparesis, brain stem signs, and peripheral neuropathies. Delirium is the most commonly seen impairment of higher functions in SLE, with changes in awareness, limited attention span, disorientation, cognitive dysfunctions, perceptual aberrations, and impaired judgment. Delusions, hallucinations, and agitation may be so prominent in some patients that a schizophreniform illness is suggested, or affective changes (either depression or elation) are so striking in others that an affective disorder is considered. In these instances, however, if the patient is cooperative, careful mental status examination often demonstrates an organic substratum of the clinical psychosis.

The organic brain disorders complicating SLE commonly occur in episodes lasting six weeks to six months, and a patient may experience several similar or different episodes. The onset of neuropsychiatric dysfunction is likely to be during the first year after the disease is diagnosed, and, in some, neuropsychiatric involvement even precedes recognition of the disease. These complications usually appear when there is evidence that the disease is worsening generally; they may appear in patients already under treatment with corticosteroids. In many patients, the neuropsychiatric complications appear to respond well to adequate quantities of steroids, and exacerbations may be seen when steroid dosage is reduced below a certain critical level. In general, the immediate prognosis for improvement in the neuropsychiatric manifestations of SLE is good, especially with the use of steroids. There is some evidence, however, that the long term prognosis is poorer for those SLE patients with neuropsychiatric involvement than for those without.

In addition to the organic psychiatric disorders, somewhere between 10 and 35 percent of patients with SLE experience functional psychiatric disorders which appear unrelated to the cerebral pathologic changes of lupus. A wide variety of clinical disorders has been described[15,18]—depression, schizophreniform disorders, neuroses, and personality disorders. Of these, depression is perhaps encountered most frequently. In some patients, the psychologic troubles antedated the lupus by many years; in others, they appear to be reactive to a chronic, disabling life-threatening disease. As might be expected, confusing combinations of functional and organic patterns are not unusual in SLE patients.

From a practical standpoint, the psychiatrist should recognize that the organic states are best treated with steroids, the functional states with standard psychiatric treatment methods. When these disorders occur concurrently, improvement in one may result in apparent improvement in others. For example, lifting of a depression in response to tricyclics or electroconvulsive therapy (ECT) may also result in amelioration of the signs of organic dysfunction.

Since almost every patient with SLE is treated with steroids, the question often arises as to whether the psychiatric changes are the result of steroid toxicity. There is rather a general consensus that this is rarely the case (although the possibility must always be considered). Episodes of psychiatric dysfunction often appear in SLE patients who are off steroids, and they often disappear with continuation or even increase in steroid dosages. Steroid toxicity is, therefore, seldom a satisfactory explanation for the psychiatric complications of SLE.

CUSHING SYNDROME

Cushing syndrome results from hyperfunction of the adrenal cortex, either as a primary dysfunction of the gland or because of excess production of corticotropin (ACTH) secondary to hypothalamic-pituitary dysfunction or ectopic production of ACTH by a nonendocrine neoplasm, e.g., oat cell carcinoma of the lung. The resulting increase in secretion of ACTH brings about the changes in fat distribution (moon facies, "buffalo hump," and truncal obesity) and skin (purplish-red discoloration, striae, and hirsutism) that characterize the appearance of patients with Cushing syndrome. In addition, patients usually complain of tiredness, easy fatigability, and muscular weakness. Hypertension and a host of laboratory changes attend the hormonal changes, but the diagnosis is usually based on the changed appearance combined with increased urinary excretion of 17-hydroxycorticoids.

Psychiatric symptoms and signs are serious in about 20 percent of patients with Cushing syndrome and are present but less severe in many others. Trethowan and Cobb[42] noted that when sizable groups of patients with this disorder are studied, "the catalog of psychiatric symptoms becomes so extended as to cover a large part of the total range of known psychiatric phenomena." Most authorities agree, however, that in Cushing syndrome depression is both the most common and the most severe neuropsychiatric complication. Indeed, about 10 percent of patients with Cushing syndrome attempt suicide. Psychotic depression in this disorder cannot be distinguished from psychotic depression unassociated with somatic illness. Less common but often even more severe management problems are the contrasting states of elation which have all the hallmarks of manic disease.

Not so frequent but often presenting severe management problems also are patients with delirious states manifested by irritability, anxiety, agitation, insomnia, illusions, delusions, hallucinations, disorientation, intellectual defects, and emotional lability with wide mood swings. The clinical picture is often one of wide variablity within even brief periods of time. Disrupted function may be so severe that schizophrenia is suspected, but careful examination usually reveals clear evidence of organic impairment. Sachar[33] emphasized that the affective illness occurring with Cushing syndrome appears purely functional whereas the schizophrenia-like pictures appear organic in origin.

In addition to these severe mental changes, many patients are said to experience lesser degrees of depression, elation, irritability, and personality changes. Cerebral cortical atrophy and ventricular enlargement have been found in a number of patients with the syndrome and in some appear to be sufficient in extent to contribute to the psychiatric picture. The etiology of this atrophy is unknown.

The mental changes due to Cushing syndrome usually abate at an unpredictable rate following correction of the adrenal cortical hyperactivity and return of hormone levels to normal. Neuroleptics may be of great help in controlling the psychiatric symptomatology until this is achieved. There is an obvious relation between the psychiatric complications of Cushing syndrome and those that follow exogenous steroid administration, but despite several decades of study the exact points where they coincide and where they diverge have not been firmly identified.

DELAYED POSTANOXIC ENCEPHALOPATHY[5,32]

Delayed neurologic reactions may follow cerebral anoxia due to a variety of causes—cardiac arrest, prolonged hypotension, carbon monoxide or other chemical poisoning, strangling or hanging, and complications of anesthesia. Typically the episode was severe enough to result in coma, but the patient awakened within 24 hours and showed little if anything to suggest residual brain damage. Then, after an asymptomatic period of 2 to 10 days (or sometimes even longer), the patient begins to manifest symptoms and signs of impaired cognition, often accompanied by withdrawal and depression. Less often, the relapse may be marked by the appearance of choreoathetosis, with or without the associated cognitive defects. Some patients then follow a downhill course, progressing to coma and death; others, after a variable period, improve and are left with differing degrees of residual impairment.

The danger for the psychiatrist is that the relapse after apparently full recovery will be mistaken for a functional disorder. The early clinical signs of relapse are often shifting or even bizarre,[25] and the condition has been mistaken for an hysterical disorder and for psychotic depression. But as Plum and associates[32] have noted: ". . . during even the first hour of delayed encephalopathy the incipient memory loss, diminished attention span, and mild but definite somatic neurologic abnormalities rule out functional psychosis."

When patients die of delayed postanoxic encephalopathy, the most commonly described pathologic change is widespread demyelination, although cavitary lesions involving the basal ganglia have also been observed. The pathogenesis of these delayed reactions is still unknown.

Plum and associates[32] noted that the delaycd reactions often appeared to follow shortly after the patient had increased physical activity. They suggested, therefore, that bed rest for 10 days after any severe acute anoxic episode might be wise as a prophylactic measure.

NARCOLEPSY[29,49]

If all patients with narcolepsy complained clearly and exactly of its characteristic tetrad of symptoms, the correct diagnosis would present few problems. Such is not the case, and there is evidence[36] that narcolepsy continues to be confused with schizophrenia and a variety of other functional psychiatric disorders, mostly because the history is so garbled that the possibility of narcolepsy is never even considered.

Narcolepsy has four classic manifestations: (1) attacks of irresistible sleep; (2) episodes of cataplexy; (3) hypnagogic and hypnopompic hallucinations; and (4) sleep paralysis. The diagnosis can be made by the presence of one or more of these symptoms; all four are present probably in no more than ten percent of narcoleptic patients. Attacks of irresistible sleep occur in virtually all, with cataplexy being the next most common and sleep paralysis the rarest.

Narcolepsy usually makes its clinical appearance in the second decade, often during a period when the patient is experiencing some sleep disturbance; other symptoms appear, if at all, several years later. There is often a positive family history.

The episodes of irresistible sleep are prone to occur during boring activities or after meals, i.e., at times when normal persons usually grow drowsy, but they may come during animated conversation, dancing, or swimming. They begin abruptly and usually last about 15 minutes but may persist several hours if the patient is not disturbed. The patient usually can be awakened easily, and he or she awakes feeling refreshed. A refractory period follows, to be succeeded by yet another period of sleep. Each day the patient may experience many such episodes which severely compromise normal daily activities. Many narcoleptic subjects complain as well of disturbed night sleep with frequent waking; others feel drowsy most of the time between sleep attacks.

Cataplexy refers to a sudden loss of muscle tone which may be localized or generalized. Drop attacks are its most severe presentation. The episodes last only a few seconds and are not accompanied by any change in level of consciousness. They are commonly precipitated by a sudden access of emotion—anger, surprise, humor, or even feelings of elation. Vivid hallucinations on awakening from (hypnagogic) or going to (hypnopompic) sleep are also common. They may be visual or auditory, often possess an intense dreamlike quality, and are frequently terrifying to the patient. The character and repetitive nature of these hallucinations may lead to the erroneous diagnosis of schizophrenia.[36] Sleep paralysis refers to episodes of generalized paralysis occurring on awakening from or going to sleep. The episodes usually last only a few seconds, although they may last longer and are often perceived by the patient as lasting longer. They too are frequently accompanied by intense fear. The paralysis can be dissipated by touching the patient or calling the patient's name.

In recent years, extensive neurophysiologic investigations have expanded our understanding of narcolepsy considerably. We have learned that most narcoleptics pass directly from waking to rapid eye movement (REM) sleep without going through the progressive stages of deepening sleep that are seen in normal subjects. REM sleep is characterized both by dreaming and by motor inhibition (sparing the extraocular muscles and thus permitting rapid eye movements with dreaming). It is hypothesized that most sleep attacks in narcolepsy are actually episodes of REM sleep and that both cataplexy and sleep paralysis are due to the motor inhibition that characterizes this stage of sleep (even though the narcoleptic patient is not asleep during the episodes of cataplexy and sleep paralysis). This explanation is not entirely satisfying, for it is known that not all sleep attacks in narcolepsy are accompanied by REM stage electroencephalographic and electromyographic patterns.

The diagnosis of narcolepsy is usually based on the history, but the physician often must ferret out the details of the symptomatology upon which the diagnosis can be established. In doubtful cases, simultaneous electroencephalographic and electromyographic recording in a sleep laboratory may prove the diagnosis. The direct transition from waking to REM sleep is characteristic of narcolepsy, but false negatives are not unusual.

The cornerstone of treatment[48] is the use of amphetamines (methamphetamine or methylphenidate) to reduce the incidence of sleep attacks. Imipramine is said to be useful specifically for the cataplexy, and minor tranquilizers may promote nocturnal sleep and help control hypnagogic hallucinations. Methylphenidate and imipramine have been used together safely in patients with both sleep attacks and cataplexy.

Treatment of narcolepsy cannot be established effectively with a recipe, because the medications of choice are not uniformly effective. Chronic use of amphetamines to control the sleep attacks results in amphetamine abuse in some patients. In addition, the amount of amphetamine needed for symptomatic relief may lead to toxicity, especially to the development of paranoid ideation. Also, narcolepsy and schizophrenia sometimes coexist in the same patient, thereby creating a psychopharmacologic dilemma. Lastly, adjusting to life with a disease that has such bizarre symptoms (and is so often misdiagnosed) is not easy, and patients are often in need of supportive psychotherapy in addition to appropriate pharmacology.

TRANSIENT GLOBAL AMNESIA[10,11,17]

This syndrome of circumscribed memory loss has been recognized as a discrete clinical phenomenon only since its description by Fisher and Adams in 1958. The disorder appears without warning and is manifested by the abrupt onset of disorientation to time and place, inability to lay down new memory traces which will last for more than a few moments, and retrograde amnesia going back usually for at least several hours but in some instances for many years. The patient usually appears perplexed and worried, is aware of and distressed by the loss of orientation and memory, and often questions those in attendance repeatedly as to what is going on or what has happened. During this time, patients may be able to perform complex motor and intellectual acts *if* they do not require short term memory or the registration of new memories. Physical and neurologic examinations are usually entirely normal aside from the mentative changes. After a time, varying from 30 minutes to several hours, the period of retrograde amnesia begins to shrink until memory is regained for events up to the beginning of the episode. All symptoms and signs of dysfunction dissipate within 24 hours or less, leaving as the only residual virtually total amnesia for the period of the episode itself.

Transient global amnesia occurs most often in the fifth, sixth, and seventh decades, more commonly in men than women. Patients usually give a history of remarkably good previous mental and physical health. No precipitating cause can be identified in most patients, although in some the onset has coincided with strenuous physical exercise. The EEG is usually normal as are other neurologic diagnostic procedures. Most patients experience only one such episode, but recurrences have been described.

The disorder is usually attributed to transiently impaired function of both hippocampi and hippocampal gyri; bilateral dysfunction is believed to be necessary for a discrete memory disturbance of this magnitude. A variety of possible causes has been suggested, a seizure disorder or transient ischemia being the most commonly raised possibilities. At the moment, no firmly established explanation exists.

Transient global amnesia must be differentiated from other episodic memory lapses due to migraine, temporal lobe epilepsy, and functional psychiatric disorders. Migraine differs from transient global amnesia in the history of previous similar episodes, the associated prodromal neurologic symptoms, and of course the occurrence of the headache itself. In memory lapses due to epilepsy, there are usually obvious changes in level of awareness, automatisms, and behavioral abnormalities.

Greater difficulty is likely to be encountered in the differentiation of memory loss due to transient global amnesia from functional psychiatric disorders. The patient with functional amnesia (1) is usually younger than the patient with transient global amnesia, (2) has prominent disorientation to person, (3) can lay down new memories during the episode even though remote memory is lost, (4) usually has the onset of memory loss when alone or away from home, and (5) often has a history of previous psychiatric dysfunction. In addition, the gradual shrinking of the period of retrograde amnesia that is seen during the recovery phase of transient global amnesia is almost never a feature of dissociative processes.

MULTIPLE SCLEROSIS[24]

Multiple sclerosis (MS) is a disseminated demyelinating disorder marked by exacerbations and remissions. It usually appears in previously healthy young adults, females more often than males. The onset is usually subacute (the symptom reaching its peak in from several hours to two days), but sudden onset is not unusual, with the symptoms becoming full blown over a few minutes and thus mimicking strokes. A variety of stresses has been described preceding the initial and subsequent episodes, but the relationship between stress and exacerbation has never been proved to be either exact or predictable. Symptoms and signs depend on the site of the demyelinating lesions, which may involve virtually any of the myelinated structures of the central nervous system. Symptoms of weakness, ataxia, visual changes, numbness, or paresthesias are most common initially.

Multiple sclerosis is characteristically marked by exacerbations and remissions spread over many years. Diagnosis rests upon the identification of symptoms and abnormal neurologic signs which can be explained only by the presence of multiple lesions affecting various regions of the central nervous system, plus the appearance of these lesions in stuttering fashion over a period of time. Cerebrospinal fluid (CSF) changes often help establish the diagnosis. Mild elevation of CSF protein and slight mononuclear pleocytosis are common, but elevation in CSF gamma globulin is the change most specifically related to MS. This may be demonstrated by an abnormal colloidal gold curve or by direct measurement of gamma globulin or IgG. Although this is the most consistent CSF abnormality seen in multiple sclerosis, the same change occurs in other neurologic disorders and thus is not pathognomonic of MS.

The etiology of multiple sclerosis is not known. Today most authorities probably consider it a disorder of the immune response of the nervous system to infection with viruses. It appears that the primary infection occurs many years before the appearance of the clinical signs of MS. The measles virus has been implicated most often but does not appear specific. With our uncertainty regarding the causes of MS, it is not surprising that no specific treatment is available.

The psychiatrist may encounter patients with multiple sclerosis at any point of their disease. When early, there is usually some uncertainty about the diagnosis, the symptoms being of such a nature that they might be explained by either neurologic or psychiatric disease. This is especially true when early symptoms such as vague paresthesias, dizziness, blurred vision, shakiness, or loss of the use of a limb are accompanied by only the slightest signs of dysfunction on neurologic examination. Such a presentation easily suggests to the physician an hysterical disorder, and the diagnostic confusion is not infrequently compounded by the appearance of genuine hysterical phenomena early in the course of MS.[1] We cannot agree with Walton's statement: "*Hysteria* can be confused with MS only through neglect to make a thorough examination of the nervous system."[44]

Uncertainty about making a diagnosis of MS is often fully justified, especially in the early predisseminated phase of the disease when neurologic abnormalities may be at best equivocal. We would advise rather that caution be observed by both neurologists and psychiatrists in the diagnosis of either multiple sclerosis or hysteria. Both should recall that no matter how bizarre the neurologic symptoms may appear, careful neurologic examination is always required.

Much rarer is the appearance of an acute, fulminating psychosis early in the course of MS,[24] either preceding, coinciding with, or following the onset of neurologic symptoms. Schizophrenic,[21] paranoid, hypomanic, depressive,[13] and confusional psychoses have all been described. Occasionally they have been so severe and disruptive that they have dominated the clinical picture for weeks or months before an exact diagnosis could be made. In these instances, the question always arises as to whether the psychosis is the result of the demyelinating lesions or whether the psychosis is coincidental with or perhaps reactive to the disease. Although cognitive losses may dominate the clinical picture early in the course of MS,[44] most case reports indicate that the psychoses described above are not primarily organic in their origin or manifestations and that they should be treated no differently from similar psychoses in patients without MS. Even ECT has been used effectively in these cases.

At the other end of the spectrum, psychiatric changes are common in patients with long-standing multiple sclerosis, although psychiatric assistance is not often sought in their management. Intellectual loss can be demonstrated in perhaps two thirds of those MS patients with long-standing disease, more commonly mild than severe, and manifested most strikingly by loss of short term memory.[23,39] Affective changes are significant in about one half, being equally divided between elevation and depression of mood. Surridge[39] noted that true euphoria is rare and that the mood alteration usually called euphoria might better be described as "cheerful complacency." Many chronic MS patients who appear cheerfully complacent on first encounter reveal significant underlying depression on fuller evaluation, thus demonstrating that the cheerful behavior is used by some to mask depression. Virtually all patients with persistent true euphoria have significant intellectual loss, and there is a close relationship between persistently elevated mood, denial of disability, intellectual loss, and severity of neurologic deterioration. Personality changes, especially increased irritability or apathy, are also common in chronic MS patients and probably are secondary to damage to the central nervous system.

On the other hand, depression, which is significant in many MS patients, has no predictable relationship to intellectual loss. Its incidence is the same in multiple sclerosis as in other chronic incapacitating diseases which do not involve the central nervous system.[39] Depression in MS thus should be considered largely functional and not the consequence of either the location or the extent of the demyelinating lesions. Treatment, therefore, should be no different from that in non-MS patients.

ENCEPHALITIS

Both the acute[20,27] and the subacute[19] viral encephalitides may present, especially at the outset, with clinical manifestations which suggest functional psychiatric disease. Although viral encephalitis is capable of mimicking functional disease, the rarity of published reports describing this phenomenon suggests that encephalitis actually is seldom mistaken for a functional psychosis, or, if such mistakes occur, that they go unrecognized. In the absence of systematic antibody studies on a large number of patients suffering initial episodes of psychiatric illness, the exact frequency with which this mistake occurs is unknown. The differential diagnosis was of little practical importance before the development of antiviral agents, but the promise that these agents hold for treating viral infections of the brain now makes correct early diagnosis essential.

Acute viral encephalitis has most often been mistaken for acute schizophrenia.[20,27] Subacute encephalitis has most often been confused with the more indolent forms of schizophrenia and with psychotic depression.[19] Capgras syndrome has also been reported to occur following encephalitis, as well as with other organic brain diseases.[28]

When encephalitis strikes patients with no history of previous psychiatric illness, even if the symptoms are confined largely to disorders of mentation, the possibility of an organic process is usually given serious consideration. When complaints of headache, malaise, incontinence, or "passing out" spells are added, the likelihood of an organic basis is increased. Even so, early diagnosis may be difficult. The changes on mental status examination typical of organicity may be absent; neurologic examination may be normal; investigation of the cerebrospinal fluid may reveal no significant changes; and the EEG may be normal (or unobtainable because of the patient's fear and agitation). Furthermore, fever and other somatic changes which usually point toward an infectious origin may be lacking. When viral encephalitis occurs in a patient with previously established functional psychiatric disturbance, distractors to the correct diagnosis are even more powerful, and the possibility of an infectious process may not even be entertained.

In the cases reported, what were the clinical features that suggested the correct diagnosis of viral encephalitis instead of functional psychosis?[45]

1. An increasing appreciation over time that the abnormalities found on mental status examination are more in keeping with an organic than with a functional disorder. What was thought to be schizophrenic blocking may be recognized as anomia, or a "word salad" as a fluent aphasia. Disorientation, initially obscured by agitation and assaultiveness, may become apparent. What appeared to be hallucination is recognized as illusion.

2. Abnormal neurologic signs that persist, worsen, or shift. Soft neurologic signs are not an unusual phenomenon in any hospitalized psychiatric patient, and their presence ordinarily does not suggest serious underlying neurologic disease. They do, however, alert the physician to the possibility of an active neuropathologic process and to the need for careful neurologic followup. Progression of these soft signs, the appearance of hard neurologic signs, or a change in pattern of neurologic dysfunction call for thorough neurologic investigation. Incontinence which persists for more than a few days despite treatment with neuroleptic medication also points to an organic process.

3. The recognition that what had been regarded as regression, with-

drawal, disinterest, and negativism actually represents impairment of consciousness. A diminution in the level of awareness is one of the most reliable signs of organicity; it is likewise one of the changes seen most consistently in encephalitis. The recognition of impaired consciousness must lead, therefore, to a search for its organic etiology.

4. Marked variability in clinical manifestations. The functional psychoses are not usually punctuated by periods free of psychotic manifestations. On the other hand, transient periods of lucidity are not unusual in viral encephalitis (or in other forms of acute diffuse encephalopathy). The occurrence of lucid periods should always suggest the possibility that an organic disorder is present.

5. Failure to improve or even worsening after treatment with amounts of antipsychotic medications that are usually therapeutic. Most patients with acute or subacute schizophreniform illnesses experience improvement in their psychotic symptoms and signs when antipsychotic agents are given in adequate quantities. When this fails to occur, the accuracy of the original diagnosis always should be questioned, and especially if other elements in the clinical presentation are incongruent. Patients with encephalitis also are often intolerant of dosages of antipsychotic drugs that usually are tolerated easily by patients with the functional psychoses—another suggestion that an organic process might be implicated.

6. Improvement with intravenous amobarbital. In a few instances, a sodium amobarbital interview may be helpful. Striking improvement points toward a functional diagnosis, whereas significant worsening points toward an organic matrix (although not of course to a specific diagnosis of encephalitis).

When encephalitis appears in the guise of a functional psychosis, the correct diagnosis will usually be achieved if the psychiatrist (1) maintains a questioning attitude toward the diagnosis when several elements in the clinical picture fail to fit together neatly; (2) carefully monitors both the mental and the neurologic status of the patient; (3) judiciously investigates the condition of the cerebrospinal fluid and the electroencephalogram and repeats these investigations when uncertainty persists; and (4) secures acute and convalescent serum for antibody titer determination when a suspicion of encephalitis persists.

INTRACRANIAL MASSES

Learning to detect brain tumors is an important objective in the training of both neurologists and psychiatrists. Important as it is, however, this is not the *raison d'être* for their neurologic training, even though the task often appears to be elevated to that position in the eyes of neurosurgeons and neuropathologists. Psychiatrists are expected, as a part of the medical care which they provide, to be able to diagnose intracranial masses when these masses are the cause of psychiatric symptoms. They should not, however, allow an unrealistic fear of missing the diagnosis of a brain tumor to dominate their neurologic thinking.

There is no question that psychiatrists sometimes fail to diagnose intracranial masses that are playing major roles in the symptomatology of their patients. Ample anecdotal evidence attests to this. The magnitude of the problem is, however, uncertain. Some investigators have found a significantly higher incidence of unsuspected intracranial tumors uncovered in mental hospital patients at autopsy than in non-mental hospital patients.[30] Others[22] have concluded that intracranial tumors are probably no more frequent in necropsies from mental hospitals than from general hospitals. There appears to be a concensus, however, that meningiomas make up a larger percentage of the intracranial tumors found in mental hospital patients than in nonmental hospital patients. There is also a suggestion that the meningiomas are more likely to encroach upon the frontal lobes in mental hospital patients than in general hospital patients. Many of these meningiomas uncovered at autopsy are small, and their role, if any, in the causation of the mental symptoms is doubtful. Tomlinson[41] stated that many are too small to have played any significant part clinically through localized, circumscribed displacement or destruction of brain tissue. Whitlock[47] recently speculated that meningiomas might effect changes in mental function through other mechanisms, but evidence to support this is lacking.

Spudis, Rogers, and Stein[37] approached the problem from another angle, studying patients who had been operated on for intracranial tumors who also had been examined by psychiatrists before the diagnosis of brain tumor was made. Of 679 patients with diagnosed intracranial tumors, 24 had been examined by psychiatrists before the tumor was identified, and 10 of these were either sent by the psychiatrists for definitive tests with a tentative diagnosis of brain neoplasm or were referred to other specialists for consideration of this diagnosis. Unfortunately, Spudis and associates did not explore in their paper the clinical details that might have helped us understand and avoid the failure by psychiatrists to discover the brain tumors in the other 14. The authors stated, however, that none of the 24 patients had been accepted as candidates for intensive psychotherapy by the psychiatrists who were consulted.

Intracranial tumors characteristically are manifested by focal neurologic symptoms and signs, headaches, vomiting, papilledema, and changes in the level of consciousness. Patients with these findings are seldom seen for psychiatric evaluations, and if they were, there is every reason to believe that psychiatrists would recognize the brain tumors as readily as other physicians. Unfortunately, patients suffering from brain tumors who are seen by psychiatrists appear with other guises, and it is these that psychiatrists must learn to identify, even though they are rare.

Patients with brain tumors who are seen by psychiatrists for evaluation usually appear with one of four clinical guises: (1) dementia;[2,22,34] (2) epilepsy with associated behavioral abnormalities;[2,22,26,37] (3) an atypical hypomanic or manic episode in a patient with no prior history of affective illness;[2,3,37] (4) an exacerbation of psychologic symptoms in a patient with previously identified psychiatric disease.[37] None of these presentations suggest specifically a diagnosis of intracranial tumor; each should suggest, however, an organic disorder, a thorough investigation of which may reveal the presence of tumor.

Today there is little excuse for failing to discover an intracranial mass when it is the cause of either presenile or senile dementia. Tumors are relatively rare causes of the syndrome of dementia (see Chap. 5). When tumors could be identified only by angiography and pneumoencephalography, procedures accompanied by both discomfort and morbidity, it was sometimes justified to forego these measures because of their low diagnostic yield in simple dementia. With the near general availability of radioactive brain scans and the widening accessibility of computed cranial tomography, however, there is now little justification for not actively pursuing a disease diagnosis in all patients with developing dementia.

Patients with epilepsy complicated by behavioral disturbances are often seen by psychiatrists (see Chap. 7). A few of these patients have an intracranial mass causing both the seizures and the aberrations of behavior. The diagnosis of tumor is not likely to be missed when both these clinical features appear de novo in adult life, because the combination points to the need for extensive neurologic investigation. Diagnostic error is more likely in long-standing cases, in which the absence of focal neurologic defects or the demonstration of negative diagnostic studies at some remote time is accepted as conclusive evidence against the presence of tumor. Even in the most chronic patients, a worsening of long-standing symptoms or the appearance of new difficulties should prompt thorough reassessment, with consideration given to repeat or more extensive diagnostic procedures.

An atypical hypomanic or manic episode sometimes results from an intracranial mass, but accurate diagnosis may be difficult, largely because the patient's euphoria, hyperactivity, and distractibility impede thorough assessment. When the patient is able to cooperate for the mental status examination, evidence of organic dysfunction is usually forthcoming. In the uncooperative patient, the possibility of an organic etiology should be suspected especially in the patient over the age of 40 who has a negative history for affective dysfunction. Appropriate diagnostic studies should be undertaken in such patients to identify a tumor or other organic pathology.

Lastly, the recognition that mental changes are due to cerebral tumor may be especially difficult in patients who have experienced significant psychiatric dysfunction previously. Unless the clinical picture is strikingly organic in nature or strikingly different from the earlier presentation, both psychiatrist and patient are likely to interpret new symptoms as an extension or revival of past problems. This is an avoidable error, but one to be avoided only by the psychiatrist's continued vigilance.

A critical reading of case reports in which brain tumors presented psychiatrically reveals just how rarely brain tumors mimic functional psychiatric disease with some degree of exactness. In a few cases (for example, the patient reported by Buchanan and Abram,[3] the patient described by Goldney,[12] and patient #3 of Hunter and associates[22]), the mimicry of functional psychiatric dysfunction was near perfect, at least early, and it would not be surprising had the correct diagnosis been missed. These cases are unusual, however, and our conclusion, prompted by these reports, is that brain tumors presenting psychiatrically almost always are accompanied by clinical features that point toward an organic etiology—if the physician will but look and see. The psychiatrist does not have to fear missing the diagnosis of brain tumor because there are no pointers to suggest that the diagnosis is not a functional disorder; the diagnosis usually is missed only if the pointers are ignored.

Tumors of the spinal cord may also be mistaken for functional psychiatric disorders.[8] Most of these tumors develop slowly, and patients may complain of pain, paresthesias, and motor difficulties for a long time before objective evidence of neurologic dysfunction appears. These patients may be referred to the psychiatrist on the assumption that their symptoms are hysterical. As with other somatic symptoms, the psychiatrist should not accept the complaints as functional in origin unless: (1) the diagnosis of a functional disorder makes good sense psychodynamically, and (2) a spinal cord mass has been ruled out by appropriate diagnostic studies (spinal cord x-rays, electromyography, and/or myelography).

REFERENCES

1. Aring, C.D.: Observations on multiple sclerosis and conversion reaction. Brain 88:663, 1965.
2. Avery, T.L.: Seven cases of frontal tumor with psychiatric presentation. Brit. J. Psychiatry 119:19, 1971.
3. Buchanan, D.C., and Abram, H.S.: Psychotic behavior resulting from a lateral ventricle meningioma: A case report. Dis. Nerv. Syst. 36:400, 1975.

4. Carney, M.W.P.: Hepatic porphyria with mental symptoms. Four missed cases. Lancet 2:100, 1972.
5. Dooling, E.C., and Richardson, E.P., Jr.: Delayed encephalopathy after strangling. Arch. Neurol. 33:196, 1976.
6. Douer, D., Weinberger, A., Pinkhas, J., et al.: Treatment of acute intermittent porphyria with large doses of propranolol. JAMA 240:766, 1978.
7. Ekbom, K.: Carbamazepine in the treatment of tabetic lightning pains. Arch. Neurol. 26:374, 1972.
8. Epstein, B.S., Epstein, J.A., and Postel, D.M.: Tumors of spinal cord simulating psychiatric disorders. Dis. Nerv. Syst. 32:741, 1971.
9. Feinglass, E.J., Arnett, F.C., Dorsch, C.A., et al.: Neuropsychiatric manifestations of systemic lupus erythematosus: diagnosis, clinical spectrum, and relationship to other features of the disease. Medicine (Baltimore) 55:323, 1976.
10. Fisher, C.M., and Adams, R.D.: Transient global amnesia. Acta Neurol. Scand. 40: Suppl. 9, 1964.
11. Fogolholm, R., Kivalo, E., and Bergström, L.: The transient global amnesia syndrome. An analysis of 35 cases. Eur. Neurol. 13:72, 1975.
12. Goldney, R.D.: Craniopharyngioma simulating anorexia nervosa. J. Nerv. Ment. Dis. 166:135, 1978.
13. Goodstein, R.K., and Ferrell, R.B.: Multiple sclerosis –Presenting as a depressive illness. Dis. Nerv. Syst. 38:127, 1977.
14. Green, J.B.: Dilantin in the treatment of lightning pain. Neurology 11:257, 1961.
15. Gurland, B.J., Ganz, V.H., Fleiss, J.L., et al.: The study of the psychiatric symptoms of systemic lupus erythematosus. A critical review. Psychosom. Res. 34:199, 1972.
16. Hatangdi, V.S., Boas, R.A., and Richards, E.G.: Posthermetic neuralgia: Management with antiepileptic and tricyclic drugs, in Bonica, J.J., and Albe-Fessard, D. (eds.): Advances in Pain Research, vol. 1. Raven Press, New York, 1976.
17. Heathfield, K.W.G., Croft, P.B., and Swash, M.: The syndrome of transient global amnesia. Brain 96:729, 1973.
18. Heine, B.E.: Psychiatric aspects of systemic lupus erythematosus. Acta Psychiatr. Scand. 45:307, 1969.
19. Himmelhoch, J., Pincus, J., Tucker, G., et al.: Sub-acute encephalitis. Behavioral and neurological aspects. Brit. J. Psychiatry 116:531, 1970.
20. Hollender, M.H., Duffy, P.E., Feldman, A.N., et al.: Encephalitis or schizophrenia? Int. Psychiatry Clin. 2:691, 1965.
21. Hollender, M.H., and Steckler, P.P.: Multiple sclerosis and schizophrenia: A case report. Psychiatry Med. 3:251, 1972.
22. Hunter, R., Blackwood, W., and Bull, J.: Three cases of frontal meningiomas presenting psychiatrically. Brit. Med. J. 3:9, 1968.
23. Jambor, K.L.: Cognitive functioning in multiple sclerosis. Br. J. Psychiatry 115:765, 1969.
24. McAlpine, D., Lumsden, C.E., and Acheson, E.D.: Multiple Sclerosis. A Reappraisal, ed. 2. Williams and Wilkins, Baltimore, 1972.
25. McEvoy, J., and Campbell, T.: Ganser-like signs in carbon monoxide encephalopathy (letter to Editor). Am. J. Psychiatry 134:1448, 1977.
26. Malamud, N.: Organic brain disease mistaken for psychiatric disorder: A clinicopathologic study, in Benson, D.F., and Blumer, D. (eds.): Psychiatric Aspects of Neurological Disease. Grune & Stratton, New York, 1975.

27. Misra, P.C., and Hay, G.G.: Encephalitis presenting as acute schizophrenia. Brit. Med. J. 1:532, 1971.
28. Nikolovsky, O.T., and Fernandez, J.V.: Capgras syndrome as an aftermath of chickenpox encephalitis. Psychiat. Opinion 15(2):39, 1978.
29. Parkes, J.D., Fenton, G., Struthers, G., et al.: Narcolepsy and cataplexy: Clinical features, treatment and cerebrospinal fluid findings. Quart. J. Med. 43:525, 1974.
30. Patton, R.B., and Sheppard, J.A.: Intracranial tumors found at autopsy in mental patients. Amer. J. Psychiatry 113:319, 1956.
31. Pilowski, I.: Psychological aspects of post-herpetic neuralgia: Some clinical observations. Br. J. Med. Psychol. 50:283, 1977.
32. Plum, F., Posner, J.B., and Hain, R.F.: Delayed neurological deterioration after anoxia. Arch. Intern. Med. 110:18, 1962.
33. Sachar, E.J.: Psychiatric disturbances associated with endocrine disorders, in Arieti, S. (ed.): Organic Conditions and Psychosomatic Medicine, Vol. IV. American Handbook of Psychiatry, ed. 2. Basic Books, New York, 1975. New York, 1975.
34. Sachs, E., Jr.: Meningiomas with dementia as the first and presenting feature. J. Ment. Sc. 96:998, 1950.
35. Schmidt, R.P., and Gonyea, E.F.: Neurosyphilis, in Baker, A.B., and Baker, L.H. (eds.): Clinical Neurology. Harper & Row, New York, 1976.
36. Shapiro, B., and Spitz, H.: Problems in the differential diagnosis of narcolepsy versus schizophrenia. Am. J. Psychiatry 133:1321, 1976.
37. Spudis, E.V., Rogers, J., and Stein, L.: The psychiatrist's management of patients with undiagnosed brain neoplasm. Southern Med. J. 70:405, 1977.
38. Stevens, H.: Meralgia paresthetica. Arch. Neurol. Psychiatry 77:557, 1957.
39. Surridge, D.: An investigation into some psychiatric aspects of multiple sclerosis. Br. J. Psychiatry 115:749, 1969.
40. Teng, P.: Meralgia paresthetica. Bull. Los Angeles Neurol. Soc. 37:75, 1972.
41. Tomlinson, B.E.: The pathology of dementia, in Wells, C.E. (ed.): Dementia, ed. 2. F.A. Davis Company, Philadelphia, 1977.
42. Trethowan, W.H., and Cobb, S.: Neuropsychiatric aspects of Cushing's syndrome. Arch. Neurol. Psychiatry 67:283, 1962.
43. Tschudy, D.P., Valsamis, M., and Magnussen, C.R.: Acute intermittent prophyria: Clinical and selected research aspects. Ann. Intern. Med. 83:851, 1975.
44. Walton, J.N.: Brain's Diseases of the Nervous System, ed. 8. Oxford University Press, Oxford, 1977.
45. Wells, C.E.: Dementia, pseudodementia, and dementia praecox, in Fann, W.E., Karacan, I., Pokorny, A.D., et al. (eds.): Phenomenology and Treatment of Schizophrenia. Spectrum Publications, Inc., New York, 1978.
46. Wetterberg, L.: A Neuropsychiatric and Genetic Investigation of Acute Intermittent Prophyria. Svenska Bokförflaget, Stockholm, 1967.
47. Whitlock, F.A.: Suicide, cancer and depression. Brit. J. Psychiatry 132:269, 1978.
48. Yoss, R.E., and Daly, D.D.: On the treatment of narcolepsy. Med. Clin. North Am. 52:781, 1968.
49. Zarcone, V.: Narcolepsy. New Engl. J. Med. 288:1156, 1973.

CHAPTER 15

NEUROLOGIC DIAGNOSTIC PROCEDURES

ELECTROENCEPHALOGRAPHY[4,7,11,14]

Electroencephalography (EEG) is probably performed in psychiatric patients more often than any other neurodiagnostic procedure. Its safety, comfort, and modest cost all contribute to its popularity. Chauvinism, too, may play some role, for the EEG is the only commonly used neurodiagnostic procedure discovered by a psychiatrist. Berger, a German psychiatrist, was the first to record rhythmic electric potentials of the human brain, probably largely due to the activity of apical dendrites, from the surface of the intact cranium. The early recognition that these normal cerebral potentials are modified by startle, concentration, and visual imagery raised hopes that electroencephalography might be a fine technique for exploring higher human cerebral functions. In this, success has been limited at least until now with the use of conventional recording methods. We agree with the statement of Kiloh, McKomas, and Osselton[4] that "from clinical, nosological and prognostic points of view, the value of the EEG in psychiatry is limited." We are considering here, however, its value to psychiatrists as they deal with potential or established organic problems, and in this limited area, the EEG is of considerable value.

Specifically, the EEG is likely to be useful to the psychiatrist when a patient's symptoms or signs suggest: (1) the possibility of a focal neurologic lesion (manifested by focal flattening or slowing of the record); (2) the likelihood of diffuse brain dysfunction, whether acute or chronic (often associated with diffuse, slow activity); and (3) the diagnosis of an episodic disorder which might be due to epilepsy (in which paroxysmal spikes, sharp waves, and slow activity may be seen). We do not insist that an EEG must always be obtained in these situations— other data sometimes are sufficient for reaching appropriate diagnostic conclusions—but the EEG can contribute to the diagnostic evaluation in all these instances.

Even though the EEG generally lacks diagnostic specificity, it is helpful particularly in several specific clinical situations. With acute or subacute alterations in the mental status, the EEG often helps in establishing the diagnosis of delirium or another encephalopathic process. When epilepsy is being considered in a patient with episodic mentative or behavioral aberrations, the EEG is indispensable. Also, there are a few unique EEG patterns which, when seen in appropriate clinical situations, are almost diagnostic.

It is probably accurate to say that the EEG of a delirious patient is always different from the EEG of that same patient in a nondelirious state.[10] Most commonly, in delirium the EEG will be marked diffusely by a reduction or absence of normal alpha rhythms with a predominance of waves within the theta and delta (clearly pathologic) range. In other patients, and probably especially in those with delirium tremens, there is a shift from alpha to faster frequencies that may suggest a state of hyperarousal. Although a shift either downward or upward in the dominant frequencies is the rule in delirium, this does not mean that a single EEG recorded during a delirium is always recognizably abnormal. A shift in alpha rhythm of 4 Hz (e.g., from 12 to 8 Hz) may result in an EEG which is still within the range of normality; in such instances, only serial recordings will demonstrate that the initial record was clearly deviant from the patient's norm. Most patients with delirium, however, have obviously abnormal EEGs. Thus the test is especially valuable in acutely psychotic patients whose differential diagnosis lies between delirium and a functional psychosis—a diffusely abnormal EEG being incompatible with a diagnosis of functional psychosis.

The EEG is indicated in virtually every patient whose mentative or behavioral abnormalities occur in well defined, brief episodes. Seizure disorders may be seen by the psychiatrist in a spectrum extending from brief staring spells with lapses in thought to longer lasting periods of disorganized or even violent behavior for which the patient is amnesic upon recovery (see Chap. 7). In such situations in which the diagnosis of epilepsy is suspected, the EEG is often the only means to confirm a diagnosis of epilepsy. An EEG with prominent paroxysmal epileptiform discharges is strong confirmation of the clinical impression of epilepsy. On the other hand, epileptic seizures are often simulated in psychiatric patients (probably largely through unconscious mechanisms), and the EEG may be useful in these patients as well. Although a normal EEG does not exclude epilepsy, an EEG that remains normal during a "spell" or even between very frequent "spells" certainly casts doubt on the diagnosis of a seizure disorder.

A single normal electroencephalogram recorded in the waking state is scant evidence against a diagnosis of epilepsy. Whenever epilepsy is considered seriously, the psychiatrist should request an EEG using conventional and nasopharyngeal leads, with the full complement of standard activating procedures—hyperventilation, photic activation, and sleep. Repeated testing is often valuable if initial records fail to reveal evidence of dysfunction.

Two conditions that may be seen initially by the psychiatrist sometimes have characteristic periodic patterns in the EEG. In Creutzfeldt-Jakob disease (subacute spongiform encephalopathy), a disease of adults due to infection with a slow virus and characterized by rapidly advancing dementia, myoclonus, and heightened startle responses, the EEG often becomes abnormal first with the appearance of periodic complexes of high amplitude sharp or triphasic waves every 0.5 to 1.5 seconds. With progression, the EEG during the interval between the periodic complexes becomes slow and then flat. No consistent correlation is found between the periodic complexes and the myoclonic jerks.

In subacute sclerosing panencephalitis (SSPE), a disease of children between the ages of 5 and 18 due to chronic infection of the brain by measles virus and characterized initially by behavioral changes and loss of intellect and later by myoclonic jerks, there is also a characteristic periodic EEG. The periodicity of SSPE differs from that of Creutzfeldt-Jakob disease in that the periodic complexes consist of two or more multiphasic delta waves appearing simultaneously and symmetrically over both cerebral hemispheres. These complexes repeat with regularity every 3 to 5 seconds. In this condition, the myoclonic jerks usually are correlated with the periodic complexes.

The EEG of the stuporous or comatose patient is usually nonspecifically abnormal, consisting of generalized slowing of the background frequencies. Rarely, however, the EEG in these patients is of such unique form that it helps to establish the cause of the stupor or coma. In hepatic coma, characteristic high amplitude and symmetrical triphasic waves in all leads are common. Electroencephalograms made up of abnormally fast background rhythms at frequencies greater than 12 to 13 Hz suggest drug overdose as the cause of the stupor or coma, and barbiturates and benzodiazopines are the usual offenders. Following anoxia and cardiac arrest, several fairly specific EEG patterns may emerge. The best known is a flat EEG, indicating absence of cerebral electrical activity. Oftentimes, however, the flat background is interrupted periodically by bursts of mixed frequency activity; this pattern is called burst suppression. An especially unusual situation is the appearance of a seemingly awake EEG in the patient who is deeply comatose. In this situation, called alpha coma, EEG activity within the alpha frequency is seen diffusely over both hemispheres, but it lacks the posterior predominance usual in the normal patient. This EEG pattern may be seen in those brain stem infarcts which disturb consciousness by interrupting the reticular formation but leave the cerebral hemispheres

225

and deep nuclei intact. This pattern may also be seen following severe anoxia. It is a poor prognostic sign.

The psychiatrist must learn to integrate the electroencephalographer's report with all of the other relevant diagnostic data. The EEG is not a precise diagnostic instrument, and the psychiatrist who treats it as such will err. The report of a "normal" EEG does not rule out organicity, and, when other data point strongly to organicity, it may be appropriate to diagnose organic disease despite the normal EEG. Equally significant, even the abnormal EEG is rarely pathognomonic of a specific organic process—indeed, petit mal epilepsy is probably the only disease that can be diagnosed unequivocally on the basis of the EEG alone. Furthermore, abnormal records are described in some 15 to 20 percent of people without recognizable neurologic or psychiatric dysfunction. The psychiatrist then must often disregard an abnormal EEG interpretation when the bulk of other evidence points away from organicity. Like all ancillary diagnostic procedures, the electroencephalogram depends on the clinician for its proper utilization.

CEREBROSPINAL FLUID[2]

As a rule, the psychiatrist should have little occasion for examination of the cerebrospinal fluid (CSF). Psychiatric patients in whom study of the CSF is essential for diagnosis are few, and although proof is lacking, most observers agree that postspinal tap morbidity (headache, nausea, back pain, malaise) is significantly greater in emotionally disturbed patients than in others. Furthermore, noninvasive diagnostic procedures now often allow the physician to reach a correct diagnosis without the necessity of spinal fluid examination. A spinal tap, therefore, should be a rare requirement among psychiatric patients and should be used only in situations in which it is likely to play some definite diagnostic or therapeutic role.

Cerebrospinal fluid findings are pathognomonic in only a few conditions: (1) infections of the central nervous system, including syphilis; (2) subarachnoid hemorrhage; (3) neoplastic involvement of the meningeal or ventricular surfaces. The latter two disorders are unlikely to be encountered in psychiatric practice. In two other specific clinical situations, examination of the CSF may be especially helpful. (1) When multiple sclerosis is suspected, elevation of the gamma globulin fraction is practically diagnostic, although its absence does not rule out the diagnosis. (2) In a setting suggesting subacute sclerosing panencephalitis (SSPE), the finding of high measles antibody titers in the CSF is virtually diagnostic. Thus for practical purposes, the psychiatrist is likely to find the CSF abnormalities of specific diagnostic assistance only in the presence of infections or multiple sclerosis.

Specifically, the psychiatrist should require CSF examination in:

1. Acutely psychotic patients whose clinical signs—change in level of consciousness, disorientation, cognitive loss, unusual findings on neurologic examination, fever, headache (clinically or historically)—suggest infection. Acute viral encephalitis may present as a fulminating psychosis with sparse evidence on neurologic examination to signal a primary neurologic disease. Acute bacterial meningitis very rarely may do the same.

2. Patients with chronic psychiatric distress who develop evidence pointing to infection (e.g., fever, leukocytosis) or neurologic changes (e.g., slight reflex asymmetry) for which there is no definite explanation. In other words, fever of unknown origin or suspicious neurologic changes call for the same thorough medical evaluation in the psychiatric as in the nonpsychiatric patient.

3. Patients with a positive serologic test for syphilis with or without previous treatment, especially if the clinical picture is compatible with a diagnosis of meningovascular syphilis, general paresis, or tabes dorsalis.

4. Patients with a history of treated or untreated syphilis (even if the serology is negative) whose clinical pattern is compatible with a diagnosis of meningovascular syphilis, general paresis, or tabes dorsalis. In these relatively rare instances, the physician should request that a treponema pallidum immobilization test and a fluorescent treponemal antibody test be performed on the CSF rather than just the routine VDRL, Kolmer, or Wasserman.

5. Patients whose history and neurologic findings suggest a diagnosis of multiple sclerosis. Strictly speaking, the CSF changes in multiple sclerosis are not pathognomonic. The CSF may remain normal even during serious exacerbations of MS, and elevated gamma globulins occur in other disorders. But when the typical clinical constellation occurs along with significant elevation in CSF gamma globulin, especially IgG (and particularly when this does not reflect a rise in the serum level of this fraction), the diagnosis of multiple sclerosis is virtually certain.

We do not suggest that CSF examination should be limited invariably to the psychiatric patients who fall into these five groups. Many other situations occur in this patient population which make study of the CSF both useful and desirable. The psychiatrist should, however, always weigh carefully what is likely to be gained by the spinal tap against its costs. It should not become a routine or casual procedure.

COMPUTED CRANIAL TOMOGRAPHY[6,8]

Computed cranial tomography (CT-scanning) "has become the initial procedure of choice in the evaluation of patients with diseases related to the brain, has virtually replaced pneumoencephalography, and has reduced the need in many instances for arteriography and radionuclide brain scanning."[5] In short, CT-scanning, within the few years of its availability, has revolutionized the radiologic investigation of brain dysfunction. As a noninvasive, safe, and painless diagnostic procedure, it has increased enormously the opportunities for psychiatrists to study patients thoroughly for possible brain lesions. Whereas in the past psychiatrists were understandably and appropriately hesitant to expose patients to the discomfort and even dangers of procedures such as arteriography and pneumoencephalography on the mere suspicion of intracranial pathology, CT-scanning makes such diagnostic completeness an everyday and necessary event.

Computed cranial tomography represents the application of sophisticated computer techniques to x-ray investigation of the head. A series of narrow x-ray beams are passed through several horizontal axes of the cranium at intervals of 1° until 180° has been traversed. Absorption of these x-ray photons is measured by a scintillation crystal rather than an x-ray film. This is converted into data which is fed into a computer which translates this information into an image displayed on a cathode ray tube or a television screen which is then photographed. The result of these manipulations is a series of pictures of the intracranial contents taken in several horizontal planes.

The images obtained by the CT-scanner vary in lightness and darkness in proportion to the attenuation or absorption of x-radiation by specific cranial and intracranial structures. Thus bones usually appear white, the ventricles filled with cerebrospinal fluid dense black. Ordinarily bone, brain parenchyma, and ventricular spaces are well delineated, as are a variety of pathologic conditions including atrophy, masses, and infarcts. When masses or vascular abnormalities are suspected, contrast enhancement, i.e., doing the CT-scan after intravenous injection of a radiopaque material to bring about better visualization of abnormal structures, is often utilized.

The radiation dose involved in computed cranial tomography is small, the skin dose of radiation being approximately the same as that from a few conventional lateral skull x-rays, and the total radiation dose to the intracranial contents is approximately one third that from a single lateral skull x-ray. Computed cranial tomography is noninvasive (unless performed with contrast enhancement), painless, safe, and usually takes no longer than 30 minutes. It remains a relatively expensive procedure, but its advantages far outweigh its cost for the psychiatric population in whom radiographic study of intracranial structures is indicated.

Woods[15] listed the main indications for computed cranial tomography in psychiatric patients: (1) a focal abnormality on neurologic examination which suggests an intracranial lesion; (2) dementia; (3) a persistent or unexplained confusional state; (4) seizures; (5) a focal or generalized EEG abnormality; (6) a history of rage attacks or impulsive aggressive behavior; (7) psychologic test findings which suggest organicity; (8) an unusual headache history. These are not, of course, the only indications—a suspicion of almost any disorder mentioned in this book might be adequate reason for referral for CT-scan. In the McLean Hospital series of psychiatric patients whose neurologic status prompted CT-scanning, 46 percent showed at least some questionable abnormality on the scan. These patients had, of course, been selected from a much larger group of patients whose psychiatric dysfunction did not suggest underlying neurologic dysfunction. On the basis of his studies, Woods[15] concluded that the CT-scan should not be used as a routine screening procedure for organicity but should be reserved for those patients (about 10 percent of inpatients in the McLean series) in whom there is specific reason to suspect organicity.

Computed cranial tomography is a new procedure, and the exact limits of its usefulness and its accuracy are not yet known. There is good evidence, however, that its judicious use significantly reduces the need for other invasive neurodiagnostic procedures which are associated with significant morbidity.[3] A "normal" CT-scan does not absolutely exclude intracranial pathology. The location of some lesions (such as craniopharyngiomas) or their small size may prevent the early recognition of some focal lesions by this procedure, and repeat scans at a later date may be required before the lesion is apparent. In other instances, clinical signs may precede the changes that would be exposed by the CT-scan. For example, in some types of dementia, changes in brain function might be expected to precede brain atrophy by a significant period. On the other hand, we have cautioned elsewhere[13] against assigning excessive significance to relatively trivial changes observed on computed cranial tomograms. When a CT-scan report does not fit the clinical picture, the accuracy and significance of the scan findings should be assessed and questioned along with the accuracy of the clinical observations. The CT-scan should be regarded by the psychiatrist as a valued guide in diagnostic evaluation and not as an exact diagnostic instrument.

OTHER RADIOLOGIC DIAGNOSTIC PROCEDURES[9,12]

Plain Skull Radiographs

Plain skull radiographs have long served as an early and basic screening procedure in patients in whom intracranial disease is suspected. The yield of diagnostically useful data is unquestionably low, and the role that the procedure should play in diagnostic evaluation deserves a critical scrutiny that cannot be provided here. Plain skull x-rays may demonstrate a variety of changes pointing to specific pathology— neoplasms, arteriovenous anomalies, metabolic diseases, trauma—but normal skull x-rays afford little assurance that the intracranial structures are free of disease.

Plain skull x-rays are probably of most specific use to the psychiatrist in cases of trauma or suspected trauma. Recent skull fractures usually are demonstrated well radiographically. The fracture line may be difficult to discern, but when a skilled radiologist is prompted to search specifically for fractures, it is likely that few pass undetected. A pineal shift may also be observed after trauma, pointing to a subdural or epidural hematoma. Plain skull radiographs are then of most specific value in ruling out recent skull fractures (fractures heal and the fracture lines disappear with time) and intracranial hematomas.

On the other hand, not every patient who has experienced head trauma requires skull x-rays. The Federal Drug Administration recently suggested[1] that, with trauma, skull radiographs should be reserved for those patients with a history of (1) unconsciousness, (2) gunshot wound or skull penetration, and (3) previous craniotomy with shunting tube in place or with examination findings of (1) skull depression, (2) discharge from ear, (3) CSF discharge from nose, (4) blood in the middle ear cavity, (5) Battle's sign (ecchymosis first appearing near the tip of the mastoid process after fracture of the base of the skull), (6) fixed dilated pupils, (7) depression of consciousness not related to alcohol ingestion, and (8) focal neurologic signs. To this we would add that plain skull radiographs are often required after head trauma for medicolegal reasons.

When indications of neurologic dysfunction are of such magnitude that more extensive neuroradiologic diagnostic procedures are perforce to be carried out, plain skull radiographs should be obtained only in cases in which they are likely to yield information of specific diagnostic or therapeutic value beyond that likely to be yielded by the other neurodiagnostic procedures.

Radioactive Brain Scan

The radioactive brain scan is based upon the capacity of certain intracranial lesions to concentrate specific radioactive substances in quantities sufficient that they can be detected by external counting devices. Usually, radioactive isotopes of mercury or technetium are injected intravenously, and scans or scintiphotos are obtained 30 to 45 minutes later. The technique is excellent for demonstration and localization of such varied lesions as neoplasm, abscess, hematoma, contusion, infarction, and vascular malformations. Although not infallible, it is nevertheless an excellent screening technique for such lesions. It cannot demonstrate brain atrophy, a significant limitation in the neuro-radiologic investigation of many psychiatric patients. With the increasing availability of computed cranial tomography, the radioactive brain scan is used much less now than only a few years ago. It remains, however, an especially valuable tool in areas where CT-scans are unavailable. It may also demonstrate certain lesions (e.g., bilateral subdural hematomas and obstruction of the venous sinuses) with greater clarity than the CT-scan usually does.

Radionuclide Cisternography

When radioactive substances are injected into the subarachnoid space at the time of lumbar puncture, their subsequent distribution throughout the subarachnoid and/or ventricular spaces can be followed by radionuclide images. Normally, the radiopharmaceutical reaches the basal cisterns in about an hour, the frontal poles and the sylvian fissure in 2 to 6 hours, the cerebral convexities in 12 hours, and the sagittal sinus area in 24 hours, by which time the substance has virtually disappeared from the basal cisterns. Absorption of the radionuclide into the blood is usually nearly complete by the end of 48 hours. The radiopharmaceutical does not normally enter the cerebral ventricles.

Several abnormalities have been observed with intracranial disease. Perhaps most common, the radionuclide may be seen to enter the cerebral ventricles in a variety of disorders associated with ventricular dilatation. Less common but possibly of more specific diagnostic importance, passage of the radionuclide over the convexities of the cerebral hemispheres, its concentration along the sagittal sinus, and its absorption there also may be impeded or absent. The latter is characteristic of normal pressure hydrocephalus which is thought to result when flow of spinal fluid through the subarachnoid spaces is blocked. The use of radionuclide cisternography is now virtually limited to the study of patients in whom a diagnosis of normal pressure hydrocephalus is suspected but has not been confirmed by other diagnostic measures.

Air Studies

For over half a century, air and other gases have been used for the opacification of the subarachnoid and ventricular spaces. When air is injected into the lumbar subarachnoid space (the most frequently used technique), the procedure is called pneumoencephalography; when the air is injected into the lateral ventricles via cannulae inserted through cranial burr openings, the procedure is called ventriculography. The latter technique is employed when evidence of increased intracranial pressure suggests lumbar puncture might be dangerous or when for one or another reason the ventricles cannot be visualized by pneumoencephalography.

Pneumoencephalography is an excellent ancillary diagnostic technique for the demonstration of atrophic processes (either diffuse or focal), masses, pituitary lesions, and congenital malformations. It provides more precise and detailed information about ventricular anatomy and patency than does any of our other diagnostic procedures. Unfortunately, pneumoencephalography is almost always attended by significant morbidity. Headache, nausea, and meningismus occur in virtually all subjects and are often severe for 24 to 48 hours. The comfort and safety of computed cranial tomography have greatly reduced our reliance on air studies even though the images provided by the CT-scan are not quite as detailed as those provided by air contrast radiography.

Cerebral Angiography

The cerebral vasculature, both arterial and venous, may be demonstrated radiographically after intra-arterial injection of radiopaque contrast media. Most frequently, the contrast media is injected directly into the major extracranial cerebral arteries (e.g., internal carotids and vertebrals) via a catheter introduced through the femoral artery and guided up to the arch of the aorta where the cerebral arteries arise. By using this approach, both the extracranial and intracranial course of these arteries may be visualized.

Cerebral angiography provides specific evidence about arterial stenosis or occlusion, aneurysms, and vascular malformations. It also allows localization of masses through display of stretching and displacement of the nearby vasculature, both arterial and venous. Inflammatory diseases involving cerebral vessels, such as systemic lupus erythematosus, may also be demonstrated. Subdural hematomas may be recognized by the appearance of a cresent-shaped avascular space between the cerebral cortical mantle and the cranium. Cerebral angiography is not very useful for demonstrating cerebral atrophy, but enlargement of the cerebral ventricles can be recognized by the stretching and displacement of the periventricular vessels.

As with pneumoencephalography, the use of cerebral angiography diminished strikingly with the advent of computed cranial tomography. It remains a valuable and required diagnostic technique, however, for the specific study of vascular lesions. As treatment of vascular diseases both before and after the occurrence of strokes improves, it is likely that psychiatrists will need to know more and more about the specific values and limitations of cerebral angiography.

REFERENCES

1. Federal Drug Administration: Selection criteria reduce unnecessary skull x-rays. FDA Drug Bulletin 8:30, 1978.
2. Fishman, R.A.: Cerebrospinal fluid, *in* Baker, A.B., and Baker, L.H. (eds.): Clinical Neurology. Harper and Row, New York, 1977.
3. Freemon, F.R., Allen, J.H., Duncan, G.W., et al.: Controlled use of cranial computerized tomography. Arch. Neurol. 35:129, 1978.
4. Kiloh, L.G., McKomas, A.J., and Osselton, J.W.: Clinical Electroencephalography, ed. 3. Appleton-Century-Crofts, New York, 1972.
5. Lowry, J., Bahr, A.L., Allen, J.H., Jr., et al. : Radiological techniques in the diagnostic evaluation of dementia, *in* Wells, C.E. (ed.): Dementia, ed. 2. F.A. Davis Company, Philadelphia, 1977.
6. New, P.F.J., and Scott, W.R.: Computed Tomography of the Brain and Orbit (EMI Scanning). Williams and Wilkins, Baltimore, 1975.
7. O'Leary, J.L., Landau, W.M., and Brooks, J.E.: Electroencephalography and electromyography, *in* Baker, A.B., and Baker, L.H. (eds.): Clinical Neurology. Harper and Row, New York, 1977.
8. Peterson, H.O., and Kieffer, S.A.: Addendum: Neuroradiology: Computed tomography of the head, *in* Baker, A.B., and Baker, L.H. (eds.): Clinical Neurology. Harper and Row, New York, 1977.
9. Peterson, H.O., and Kieffer, S.A.: Neuroradiology, *in* Baker, A.B., and Baker, L.H. (eds.): Clinical Neurology. Harper and Row, New York, 1977.
10. Pro, J.D., and Wells, C.E.: The use of the electroencephalogram in the diagnosis of delirium. Dis. Nerv. Syst. 38:804, 1977.
11. Solomon, S.: Electroencephalography, *in* Freedman, A.M., Kaplan, H.I., and Saddock, B.J. (eds.): Comprehensive Textbook of Psychiatry, ed. 2. Williams and Wilkins, Baltimore, 1975.
12. Taveras, J.M., and Wood, E.II.: Diagnostic Neuroradiology, ed. 2. Williams and Wilkins, Baltimore, 1976.
13. Wells, C.E., and Duncan, G.W.: Danger of overreliance on computerized cranial tomography. Am. J. Psychiatry 134:811, 1977.
14. Wilson, W.P. (ed.): Applications of Electroencephalography in Psychiatry. A Symposium. Duke University Press, Durham, N.C., 1965.
15. Woods, B.T.: CT scanning in an adult psychiatric population. McLean Hosp. J. 1:150, 1976.

INDEX

Gilles de la Tourette syndrome
 course of, 174-175
 definition of, 174
 treatment of, 175
Glabella tap reflex, eliciting of, 39
Graphesthesia, 28
 testing for, 35-36
Grasp reflex, eliciting of, 37

HABIT spasms. *See* Tics.
Hallucinations, narcoleptic, 211
Hallucinosis, alcoholic, 133-134
Headache. *See also* Facial pain.
 definition of, 97
 depression and, 103-104
 functional, 102-103
  treatment of, 108
 intracranial lesions and, 105
 meningeal irritation and, 105
 migraine. *See* Migraine.
 muscle contraction, 101-102
 nonrecurring, 104-105
 orgasmic, benign, 101
 post-traumatic, 104-105
 psychiatric evaluation of, 112-113
 recurring
  depressive, 103-104
  nasal sinus obstruction, 102
  nonvascular
   functional, 102-103
   hypertensive, 102
   muscle contraction, 101-102
   treatment of, 107-108
  vascular. *See* Migraine.
 structures giving rise to, 97
 temporal arteritis and, 104
 treatment of, 105-108
Head trauma
 dementia following, 194-195
 personality changes following. *See*
  Episodic dyscontrol; Frontal lobe
  syndrome.
 post-traumatic amnesia with, 193, 194
 psychoses following, 194
 retrograde amnesia with, 193
Hemifacial spasm
 course of, 169
 etiology of, 169-170
 treatment of, 170
Herpes zoster
 course of, 205
 etiology of, 205
 of gasserian ganglion, 110-111
 incidence of, 206
 symptoms of, 206
 treatment of, 206
Histamine cephalgia, 100
Hoffmann sign, testing for, 30
Hoover's sign, 24

Horton's headache, 100
Huntington chorea
 dementia in, 173
 treatment of, 174
Hydrocephalus, normal pressure, 231
Hyperosmolality, nonketotic, delirium
 and, 60
Hyperreflexia, symmetrical, bilateral, 36
Hyperthermia, in delirium, 60
Hypoglycemia
 delirium and, 60
 syncope, and, 158
Hyporeflexia, symmetrical, bilateral, 36
Hyposexuality, epileptic, 123-124
Hypothermia, in delirium, 52
Hysteria, delirium distinguished from, 56

INTERMITTENT porphyria, acute
 diagnosis of, 204
 presentation of, 203
 treatment of, 204
Intracranial masses
 diagnosis of, 217-218
  difficulties in, 219-220
  techniques in, 219
 presentations of, 219

KINESEGENIC choreoathetosis,
  paroxysmal, 175-176
Kleine-Levin syndrome, 74
Korsakoff syndrome. *See also* Wernicke
  syndrome.
 amnesia in, 138
 clinical features of, 138
 confabulation in, 138
 insight deficiency in, 138-139
 intellectual capacity in, 139
 prognosis in, 139

LANGUAGE function, psychiatric
  evaluation of, 11-13
Locked-in syndrome, 73-74

MARCHIAFAVA-BIGNAMI disease, 139
Ménière disease, 162
Meningiomas, studies of, 218
Mental status examination
 consciousness level in, 7
 intellectual evaluation in
  conceptualization in, 10
  constructional abilities in, 13-14
  general knowledge assessment in, 9
  language function in, 11-13
  numerical skills in, 10
  problem-solving ability in, 10
  proverb interpretation in, 10
  situational understanding in, 10-11
 memory evaluation in, 8-9
 mood assessment in, 14